DENISE MARKS, M.D.

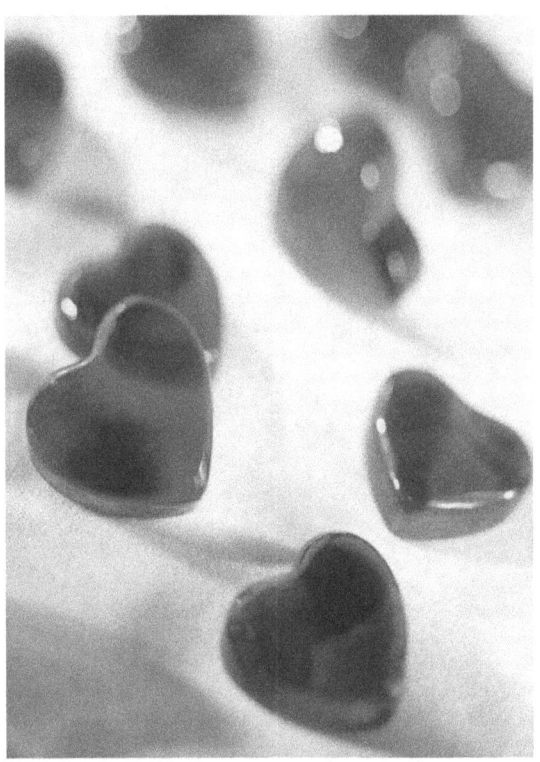

THE IMPORTANCE OF THE "SUGAR/FIBER" RATIO!

THE IMPORTANCE OF THE "SUGAR/FIBER" RATIO!

Is sugar good for you?

Generally Not! Only natural sugars found in fruits, grains and vegetables are considered necessary and healthy. These natural sugars are carbohydrates that contain phytonutrients such as antioxidants & anti-inflammatories as well as fiber.

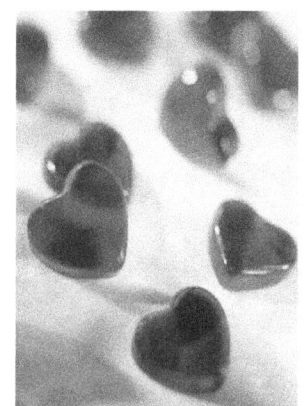

It is now known that the over consumption of sugar is not healthy. In fact, consuming 90 grams (equivalent to 2 medium soft drinks) of added sugar daily can cause many of the modern-day metabolic (inflammatory) diseases.

Furthermore, added sugar contains empty calories. Empty calories simply means that foods sweetened or made with sugar (like candy, cookies, cereals, salad dressings, sugar flavored water, juices, teas, coffee, and so many other processed foods) have little or no nutritional value. And the nutritional value of carbohydrates verses the risk of causing diseases can be somewhat determined by either the sugar/fiber ratio, carb/fiber ratio or the carb/sugar ratio. But the simplest and most useful marker that determines the nutritional value of these foods that contain carbohydrates is - the "sugar/fiber" ratio.

THE IMPORTANCE OF THE SUGAR/FIBER RATIO

Please direct online inquiries to:

admin@atozpublishinggroup.com or thormahlen46@gmail.com.

For written inquiries:

AtoZ Publishing Group, LLC
40 Plaza Way, 8-132, Mountain Home, AR 72653

http//www.atozpublishinggroup.com
http//denisesharbono.atozpublishinggroup.com

First AtoZ Printing September 2014
Published in the United States of America

Other Books by

Denise Marks, M.D.

God's Amazing Pharmacy

Food Is Your Best Medicine

A Great Nation & A Company of Nations

Table of Contents

INTRODUCTION -- IS SUGAR GOOD FOR YOU?

Is sugar good for you? Generally Not! Only natural sugars found in fruits, vegetables, grains nuts and seeds are considered necessary and healthy. That is because these natural sugars are carbohydrates that contain fiber as well as important phyto-nutrients such as antioxidants and anti-inflammatory micronutrients.

It is well known that the over consumption of sugar (90 grams of added sugar or more a day) is considered <u>not</u> healthy. In fact this amount of sugar is now known to cause (trigger) many of our modern-day, inflammatory, metabolic diseases.

Furthermore, added sugar contains empty calories. Empty calories simply means that when you eat foods sweetened with sugar (like candy, cookies, cereals, salad dressings, sugar flavored water, juices, teas, coffee, and so many other processed foods) you are consuming food with little or <u>no nutritional value per calorie</u>.

 The <u>nutritional value</u> of sugar containing foods (i.e., simple and complex carbohydrates) <u>versus the risk of causing diseases</u> can be determined by either the <u>sugar/fiber</u> ratio, <u>carb/fiber</u> ratio or the <u>carb/sugar</u> ratio. But **the simplest and most useful marker that determines the nutritional value of these foods is simply - the "<u>sugar/fiber</u>" ratio.**

Several guide lines have been established by scientists to determine the nutritional value of foods that contain carbohydrates. Again, these guide lines are based on the <u>sugar/fiber</u> ratio, the <u>carb/fiber</u> ratio and/or the <u>carb/sugar</u> ratio.

However, the simplest and most useful marker that determines the nutritional value of food that contains carbohydrates is - the "<u>sugar/fiber</u>" ratio. Basically, all three of these ratios indicate the amount of fiber contained in any carbohydrate (food). **And it is the**

1

Denise Marks, M.D.

amount of fiber in these carbohydrates that often determines their nutritional value.

Also, it is the amount of fiber in carbohydrate foods that determines their glycemic value. For example, carbohydrates that contain lots of fiber grams per sugar grams would be considered a healthy, low glycemic choice and a carbohydrate that contains very little fiber grams per sugar grams would be a unhealthy, high glycemic choice and thus would be less nutritious and more likely to cause one or more of the well known modern-day inflammatory metabolic diseases.

 Some of these well known inflammatory metabolic diseases are: diabetes, nearly all vascular diseases such as hypertension, atherosclerosis, heart and kidney diseases, eye diseases, gastro-intestinal diseases such as Crohn's and irritable bowel problems, skin diseases, arthritis, some neurological and anxiety or nervous diseases and even some cancers.

The important issue to remember is that consuming foods with a higher percentage of fiber than the percentage of sugar will provide a more nutritionally dense choice and therefore a healthier food choice.

For example, 100 calories of unsugared strawberries is healthier than

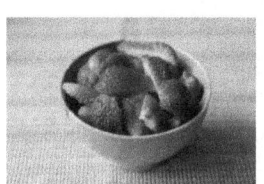

100 calories of sugared sweetened strawberries. Unsugared strawberries provide more healthy nutrients as well as fiber per calorie and are therefore said to be more nutritionally dense. Also, the unsweetened strawberries' sugar/fiber ratio as well as the glycemic index is lower and therefore better than the sugar sweetened strawberries.

However, the main reason to be interested in the sugar/fiber ratio (or the glycemic value) of any carbohydrate is that sugar and fiber

2

have <u>contrasting roles</u> after consumption as well as during the metabolism of that food. (<u>Note</u>- <u>Metabolism is the chemical breakdown of food during digestion and the usage of these food nutrients once they are absorbed into the blood stream</u>).

Simple carbohydrates that contain very little fiber (monosaccharides) are rapidly absorbed from the digestive tract which then raises the blood sugar level abruptly and rapidly. This abrupt - rapid rise - in the blood sugar level causes a surge of insulin to be poured into the circulation.

Now you have an abnormally high level of both sugar (glucose) and insulin in the blood stream. This higher than normal level of glucose (sugar) and insulin in the circulatory system is what is now known to trigger most of our modern-day inflammatory, metabolic, diseases.

Note- fiber slows the absorption of sugars - which means fiber slows the rate of rise in the blood sugar level and therefore prevents a surge or an abrupt rise in the blood insulin level.

During exercise when the body needs a lot of energy quickly, a low fiber sweet drink will cause a rapid rise in blood sugar but <u>this level of sugar will be used up quickly</u> by the cells - for energy. The real trouble begins when one lives a more sedentary life style.

For example, when we consume low-fiber sweet drinks (colas and processed juice drinks) that contain an <u>excess of sugar compared to the amount of fiber</u> and the sugar is not used up quickly then this <u>excess sugar gets converted into fat</u> (Note- <u>triglycerides</u> is another name for <u>fat</u>).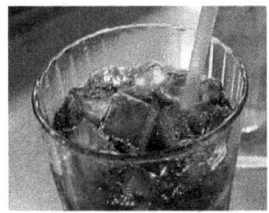

Another way of stating this concept is: when the overall <u>energy supply</u> (food) is high (especially from added sugar or processed high fructose sugar drinks) and <u>utilization</u> is low (sedentary lifestyle) as

3

with the current American or Western lifestyle and diet, <u>the blood sugar is not used for energy as fast as it is being absorbed</u>. And any excess blood sugar is converted to fat (i.e., triglyceride molecules) in and by the <u>liver</u>. Once glucose is converted into fat molecules (triglyceride molecules), many of these triglyceride molecules are put into the circulation to be delivered to fat cells for storage. This causes hyperlipidemia, high blood pressure which will lead to heart disease and several other inflammatory vascular diseases.

Also, many of the sugar laden soft drinks and processed juice drinks, especially the ones containing <u>high fructose corn syrup</u>, are more likely to be deposited as fat in the liver: causing what is known as a <u>fatty liver syndrome</u>. This would happen even if that person does not consume fatty foods and is on a vegetarian diet.

Note- <u>Fat production and storage</u> is as much related to the pace at which sugars are absorbed into the blood stream as it is the overall amount of sugar in a given meal. And that is where or when fiber becomes an important part of the metabolic process, as fiber slows down the rate at which sugar is absorbed.

Remember: <u>Two foods can be eaten with identical calories and grams of sugar, yet the result in patterns of usage </u>(energy versus fat production) <u>is very different</u> - and it all depends on the <u>sugar/fiber ratio</u> or the amount of fiber in that particular amount or type of food. <u>When adequate fiber exists in the meal, that fiber slows down the absorption of sugars</u>. When the blood sugar rise is spread over a longer time interval it allows the food to become metabolized for energy (used by the cells for energy) instead of stored as fat. The net result is that none or very little sugar will be converted to fat (triglycerides).

Also note, just as important as the amount of and/or rate of sugar that is absorbed, is the <u>surge or amount of insulin </u>that is released into the blood stream. Studies indicate that the <u>plasma (blood) insulin</u>

levels are significant independent predictors of the productions of low density lipoprotein (LDL) as well as cholesterol production, heart disease, diabetes and weight gain.

Technically, it is not the availability of triglyceride or free fatty acid (FFA) that determines the production of low density lipoproteins (LDL) as well as the amount of body fat or the distribution of body fat that is stored: but rather it is the amount of sugar and insulin, together, that chronically remains high throughout the day that determines the production of low density lipoproteins (LDL) and the amount as well as the distribution of body fat that is stored.

Another way to explain what this information means is that the production or cause of LDL (low density lipoproteins), cholesterol, heart or vascular disease and the many other inflammatory diseases is based on the amount of chronically high glucose (sugar) and insulin levels in the blood stream.

These two agents of inflammation play a greater role in causing the modern day metabolic diseases. And a better way to test for the risk of heart disease and hypertension as well as most of the modern-day inflammatory metabolic diseases is to measure a two (2) hour - post-prandial blood level of both glucose and insulin as well as LDL-cholesterol and triglyceride (TG) levels. The numerical information gathered from this test indicates how well the body can utilize carbohydrates, especially the simple carbohydrates like sugar.

Denise Marks, M.D

THE SUGAR/FIBER RATIO, CARB/FIBER RATIO, CARB/SUGAR RATIO!

The Sugar/Fiber Ratio

In order to calculate the sugar/fiber ratio of packaged foods, you will need to look at labels. The following table lists the three basic food groups found on food labels (fruit, vegetables and grains) that contain natural carbohydrates.

The following table gives the "nutritional facts" found on most food labels and these facts can be used to calculate the sugar/fiber ratio.

Label	Apple	Spinach	Whole Wheat
Carbohydrates	18 gms	1 gm	90 gms
Sugar	12 gms	0.5 gm	1 gms
Fiber	3 gms	1 gms	15 gms
Sugar/fiber ratio	4 = 4 to 1	1/2 = 1 to 1/2	1/15=1 to 15

This table applies to foods that contain only natural carbohydrates: that is - they contain no added sugar. Note- It is much more difficult to calculate the sugar/fiber ratio if the product contains artificial nonnutritive sweeteners.

By using the above data we can calculate the "sugar/fiber" ratio for an apple by dividing the grams of sugar by the grams of fiber. In the above table, under apple, sugar is 12 grams and fiber is 3 grams: so 12 divided by 3 is 4.

The sugar/fiber ratio is often stated as 4 to 1, but most nutritionists would just express this sugar/fiber ratio as 4 (four). Again using the above referenced table for spinach, the sugar/fiber ratio for spinach

6

would be the 0.5 grams of sugar divided by the 1 grams of fiber which would be ½. Spinach's sugar/fiber ratio is 1/2 to 1 or 1/2 (one-half). The sugar/fiber ratio for whole wheat would be 1 to 15 or 1/15 (one fifteenth). And this (1/15th) would be the best sugar/fiber ratio of the above.

The Carb/Fiber Ratio

The carb/fiber ratio is a different measurement for expressing the nutritional value of food. In order to calculate the carb/fiber ratio using the above referenced table of nutritional facts you will need to pick out the values for carbohydrates and fiber.

 The carbohydrate content for a single serving of an Apple, Spinach and Whole Wheat or Quinoa grains is 18 gms, 1 gm, 90 gms and 40 gms and the fiber content for that same serving is 3 gms, 1 gms, 15 gms and 5 gms, respectfully.

Carbohydrates	18 gms	1 gm	90 gms
Sugar	12 gms	0.5 gm	1 gms
Fiber	3 gms	1 gms	15 gms
Carb/fiber ratio	6= 6 to 1	1= 1 to 1	6=6 to 1

The carb/fiber ratio of the above references carbohydrates is as follows. Apple's carb/fiber ratio would be 18 divided by 3 which equals 6 to 1 or 6. Spinach's carb/fiber ratio would be 1 divided by 1 which is 1 to 1 or 1. Whole Wheat's carb/fiber ratio would be 90 divided by 15 which is 6 to 1 or 6.

Note- The carb/fiber ratio as well as the carb/sugar ratio can be used to estimate the "wholeness" of that grain product in cereal or breads. A low carb/fiber ratio means a lot more fiber per carbohydrate and therefore that food has more whole grain goodness: that is because the sugar content of that carbohydrate is

Denise Marks, M.D.

low and the fiber content is high: and therefore this product would be a better choice.

For instance, if a product contains 40 grams of carbs (carbohydrates) and 5 grams of fiber then to calculate that ratio divide 40 by 5 and you get - the <u>carb/fiber</u> ratio of 40/5 or **8**: the whole number 8 means there are 8 grams of carbohydrates for every 1 gram of fiber in that serving. **Any <u>carb/fiber</u> ratio less than 10 is considered good**. On the other hand, a <u>carb/fiber</u> ratio of 23 is considered not good. The whole number, 23, means that that food contains 23 grams of carbs for every 1 gram of fiber.

The carb/sugar ratio --can be used to determine the amount of sugar that has been added.

The carb/sugar ratio can also be used to determine the nutritional value of foods. This ratio is <u>used more to determine the amount of sugar that has been added to the carbohydrate</u>. Another way of stating this concept is that the <u>carb/sugar ratio</u> is used to determine what percentage of the carbohydrate is whole grain compared to that which is due to added sugar.

The "<u>carb/sugar</u>" ratio, which is indicative of the percentage of sugar added, is different than the <u>carb/fiber</u> ratio as well as different than the <u>sugar/fiber</u> ratio. Remember, the <u>carb/sugar</u> ratio is more indicative of the <u>amount of added sugar</u> that is in that food product.

And the difference between the total grams of carbs and the total grams of sugar <u>is more indicative of how much sugar was added in the processing of that food product</u>. For example, if the grams of carbs is 50 and the grams of added sugar is 25 then the carb/sugar ratio is <u>2</u>. And if the grams of carbs is 50 and the grams of added sugar is 5 then simply divide 50 by 5 and the carb/sugar ratio is <u>10</u>. Basically, a higher the <u>carb/sugar ratio</u> whole number is (10 is better that 2) means that food contains more whole grain and less added sugar.

TYPES OF SUGARS AND STARCHES

Sugar comes in several forms. These forms range from everyday, familiar forms to less known ones. The basic forms include:

1) Granulated sugar. This is the type of sugar most people are familiar with: the white sugar granules found in kitchens everywhere. This type of sugar is used to sweeten beverages (tea, coffee, drink mixes, etc.) and to add a sweet taste to baked or cooked goods (cookies, desserts, etc.) Sugar granules are also used to preserve jams and candied fruits.

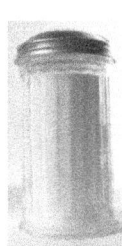

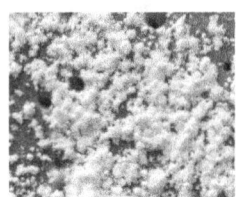

2) Powdered sugar. (Also known as milled sugar.) Fine powdered sugar is often found in confectionary creations of all types. Its most common uses include as a dust sprinkled on foods or as a glaze drizzled or spread over food.

3) Decorative sugar (aka sprinkles.) Sugar crystals are available in various colors for use in decorating foods. They can also be added to baked products or used in other confectionary creations.

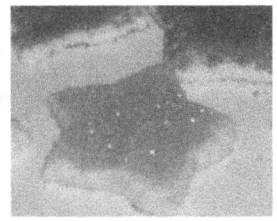

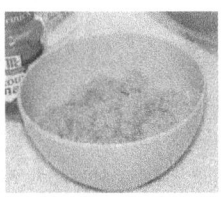

4) Brown sugar. Brown sugar is simply granulated sugar that has been coated in molasses. This type of sugar is often used in cookie, dessert, candy and confectionary recipes.

5) Cubed sugar. White or brown sugars are pressed together to create square cubes for use in confectionary creations or to sweeten beverages.

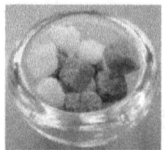

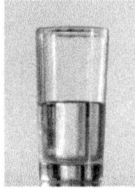

6) Liquid sugar. Sugar is dissolved in water to make syrups for use in various foods. These syrups tend to be about 67% sugar.

7) Invert sugars. This type of sugar product is actually blended according to the directions of the manufacturer that will be using the product. Found in products including bakery products, breads and beverages, invert blends are used for sweetening and moistness.

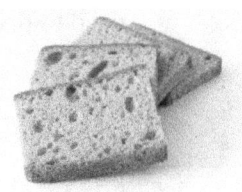

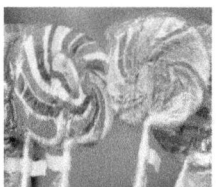

8) Syrup and treacle sugar. When inverted sugars are dissolved by heating them up, they become syrups which are then used in baked goods and candies. If molasses is added to the syrup, the result is treacle.

9) Fruit sugar. The sugar from fruit is often fermented so that it becomes alcohol. If additional sugar is added to increase the alcohol content, the process is called capitalization. In order to create a sweet wine, the fermentation process may be cut short.

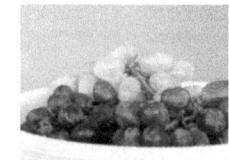

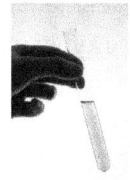

10) Maltodextrin sugar. Maltodextrin sugar is actually a synthetic, or created, sugar. It consists of short chains of glucose models and is created when starch is partially hydrolyzed. You'll find Maltodextrin listed in the contents on the label of many low calorie sweeteners.

11) Polyol sugar. Polyols are actually sugar alcohols. They're found in chewing gum and are used to prolong the flavor of the gum.

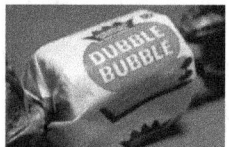

TYPES OF SUGAR STARCHES (also known as STARCH SUGARS)

STARCH SUGARS. Starch can be hydrolyzed into simpler carbohydrates by acids, various enzymes, or a combination of the two. The resulting fragments are known as dextrins. The extent of conversion is typically identified by dextrose equivalent (DE). DE is determined by the fraction of the starch bonds (glycosidic) that have been broken.

These starch sugars are by far the most common starch based food ingredient and are used as sweetener in many drinks and foods. They include:

Maltodextrin, a lightly hydrolyzed starch product used as a bland-tasting filler and thickener.

Glucose syrups, also called corn syrups in the US, viscous solutions used as sweeteners and thickeners in many kinds of processed foods.

Dextrose is commercial glucose, prepared by the complete hydrolysis of starch. Dextrose is usually used for IV therapy in hospitals

Denise Marks, M.D.

High fructose corn syrup is made by treating dextrose solutions (a solution of hydrolyzed starch) with the enzyme glucose isomerase, until a substantial fraction of the glucose has been converted to fructose.

In the United States, sugar (sucrose) prices are two to three times higher than in the rest of the world, which makes high fructose corn syrup significantly cheaper, so that it is now the principal sweetener used in processed foods and beverages. High Fructose Corn Syrup also has better microbiological stability. Note- One kind of high fructose corn syrup, HFCS-55, is sweeter than sucrose because it is made with more fructose, while the sweetness of HFCS-42 is on par with sucrose.

Sugar alcohols, such as maltitol, erythritol, Sorbitol, mannitol and hydrogenated starch hydrolysate, are sweeteners made by reducing sugars.

Modified starches: A modified starch is a starch that has been chemically modified to allow the starch to function differently under conditions frequently encountered during processing or storage, such as high heat, low pH, freeze/thaw.

PRODUCTION OF SUGARS AND STARCHES (SACCHARIDES)

PRODUCTION OF GLUCOSE BY THE LIVER

Sugar can be internally and is made - from body fat (triglycerides) - during a "fast". The internal production of glucose (sugar) from body fat (triglycerides) occurs in the **liver** during a process known as gluconeogensis. This internal production of glucose (sugar) occurs only when glucagon is produced and released from the delta cells of the pancreas which only occurs automatically during a dietary fast or long periods of strenuous activity.

When the glucose (sugar) level is low in the blood stream, then the Insulin level in the blood stream is low. When both the glucose and insulin levels are low, then and only then does the pancreas release "Glucagon", the fat burning hormone, into the blood stream. Glucagon then goes to the fat cell and triggers an enzyme that will cause the fat cell to release its stored fat, i.e., triglycerides, into the blood stream and then through a transport protein, glucagon initiates the transport of these fat molecules to the liver where this fat, (triglycerides), is converted to glucose. This chemical process is called gluconeogensis and occurs only in the liver.

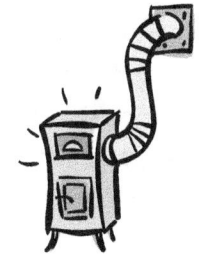

The Fat burning furnace is a term I coined to illustrate gluconeogensis. **Gluconeogensis** is the biochemical process where fat is converted to glucose (the "fat burning" process) by a series of oxidative steps. Interesting, is the fact that the diabetic medicine, "Metformin (Glucophage)" as well as alcohol, blocks this fat burning process, (gluconeogensis), in

Denise Marks, M.D.

the liver and thus lowers the glucose level in the blood stream but raises the triglyceride and cholesterol levels in the blood stream. It is easy to see that Metformin (Glucophage) lowers the blood level of glucose at the expense of raising triglyceride and cholesterol levels.

PRODUCTION OF SUGAR FROM BEETS

The sugar beet (Beta vulgaris) tuberous root contains a high quantity

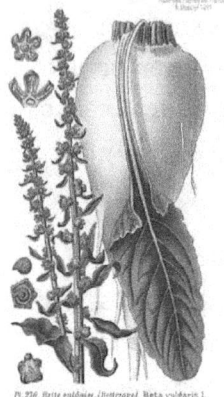

of sucrose. The plant grows in temperate regions where fertile soil and adequate rainfall are available.

Sugar beets are harvested in the fall using machinery. Since the roots do not decay quickly, it is possible to leave them in clumps in the field for some time before taking them to the processing facility. Excess soil and the leaves are removed before the beets are transported.

Upon arrival at the facility, the roots are washed and sliced so the juice can be extracted. The juice is mixed with milk of lime then carbonated in several stages for purification. The syrup is boiled in a vacuum in order to evaporate the water from it. Once cooled, the syrup crystallizes. When the crystals have dried, they are ready for use.

PRODUCTION OF SUGAR FROM SUGARCANE

Sugarcane (Saccharum spp.) is actually a perennial grass grown in tropical and subtropical regions. The plant requires a frost-free environment and adequate rainfall to make use of its excellent growth potential.

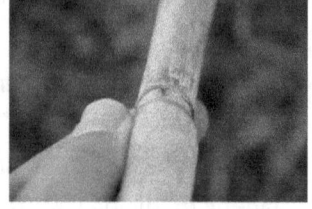

The plant can be harvested with machines or by hand. Taken quickly to the processing plant, the sugar is extracted with water or by diffusion. Lime is added and the liquid is heated to destroy enzymes. This leaves thin syrup which is further concentrated by evaporating out more water via vacuum container evaporation systems.

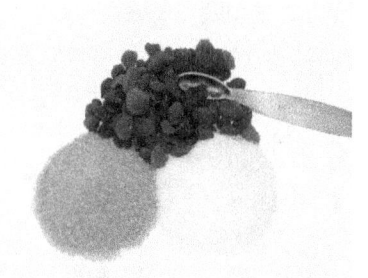

The process results in sugar crystals which must be dried out prior to use. Used as they are, the raw crystals have a brown coating. Bleached or treated with carbonation, they become whiter. Molasses is a by-product of the whitening process.

Cane sugar requires further processing to provide the free-flowing white table sugar consumers are accustomed to using.

The first stage is to remove the sticky brown coating from the crystals. During this process, impurities are removed along with precipitated particles. Once the brown coating is gone, the sugar syrup is boiled to make it concentrated. It is then cooled. The white sugar crystals are dried, making them ready to use. The surplus liquor that is spun out is made into refiners' molasses.

PRODUCTION OF SUGAR FROM STEVIA PLANT EXTRACTS

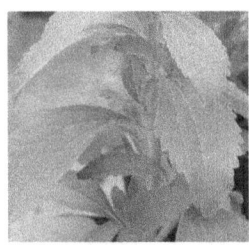

Stevia is a natural sugar. However Stevia has a slightly different taste than beet or cane sugar. Stevia actually refers to a genus of about 240 species of herbs and shrubs in the sunflower family (Asteraceae), native to subtropical and tropical regions. The species Stevia rebaudiana, commonly known as sweet-leaf, sugar-leaf, or simply Stevia, is widely grown for its sweet leaves.

Denise Marks, M.D.

As a sugar, Stevia's taste has a slower onset and longer duration than that of sugar, although some of its extracts may have a bitter or licorice-like aftertaste at high concentrations. An extract of Stevia, i.e., steviol glycoside, is more than 300 times sweeter than granulated sugar.

With the rise in demand for low-carbohydrate, sugar - sweeteners, Stevia has attracted the attention of dieters as well as producers Because <u>Stevia has a negligible effect on blood glucose</u> it is also attractive to people on low carbohydrate-controlled diets

THE PRODUCTION OF HIGH FRUCTOSE CORN SYRUP

There is a real difference between high-fructose corn syrup and the fructose that is in fruit. <u>High fructose corn syrup is made using corn starch</u> which does contain glucose, just in a different ratio than table sugar. The idea for using high-fructose corn syrup is that it doesn't dry out the same way that cane sugar does, and it's a "nifty" excuse for planting lots of corn, selling lots of seed and fertilizer and tractors, creating a new commodity for hedge funds, and so on.

<u>One of the primary sources of calories for Americans is "sugar", and more specifically -the excess sugars that come from high fructose corn syrup (HFCS)</u>. In today's world, High Fructose Corn Syrup (HFCS) is really the type of <u>starch sugar</u> most commonly used in place of granulated sugar, i.e., Sucrose.

High Fructose Corn Syrup is contained in nearly all sodas and processed foods found in our modern day super markets. This is basically done by those who process the foods for markets and it is done in order to extend the shelf life of processed drinks and processed food as well as for financial gain.

Because of advances in food processing technology in the 1970s, high fructose corn syrup derived from corn starch has become very cheap as well as HFCS extends the shelf life of processed foods.

16

THE PRODUCTION OF STARCHES

Plants produce glucose from carbon dioxide during photosynthesis. That glucose, in the form of starch granules, is stored in the plant. As the growing season winds down, starch accumulates in fruit, seeds, rhizomes and tubers. This stored starch is one of the ways the plant prepares for the next growing season.

Starch from foods, "food starch" is the most common carbohydrate in the human diet. It is found in many common foods. Worldwide, the major sources of starch are cereals (wheat, rice, maize) and root vegetables (potatoes and tapioca).

Some starchy foods are specific to certain climates. (Acorns, tapioca, arrowroot, etc.) Commonly used prepared foods containing starch include bread, pancakes, pasta and tortillas.

PRODUCTION AND TYPES OF ARTIFICAL SWEETENERS (i.e., SUGAR SUBSTITUES)

Food producers use sugar substitutes to reduce calories and to extend the shelf life of foods. Sugar substitutes can be made from natural products (Sorbitol, xylitol) or from products created artificially in a lab (aspartame, saccharin).

While it is easy to assume that non-calorie sweeteners promote weight loss, the truth may differ. Some studies have found that drinking diet soda contributes to obesity and metabolic syndrome.

> *Note- experiments have found that using artificial sweeteners in rats resulted in increased calorie intake and increased body weight.*

The results of one study suggest that consuming products that contain artificial sweeteners may lead to weight gain and obesity due to interference of physiological process that are reconciled by taste receptors. Artificial sweeteners are also known to affect hormone balance, vital to preventing metabolic diseases.

The Food and Drug Administration in the United States has approved several non-calorie sweeteners. These include aspartame, saccharin and neotame.

COMMON ARTIFICIAL SWEETENERS

Artificial sweeteners are frequently referred to as non-calorie sweeteners. This is not necessarily true. There are calories in non-calorie sweeteners. Most non-calorie sweeteners contain dextrose and/or Maltodextrin, added to provide bulk.

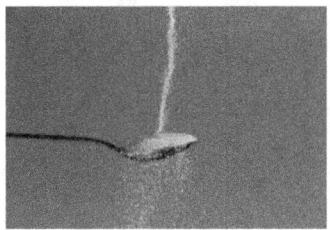

Unfortunately, both dextrose and Maltodextrin are digestible carbohydrates that add calories. Consider Sweet'N Low, Equal and Splenda. 10 grams of these sweeteners contain 33 to 36 calories, compared to 39 calories for sugar.

Based on weight, these sweeteners serve to reduce the number of calories by only ten to fifteen percent when compared to sugar. That is not a significant amount.

However, these substitute sweeteners actually allow sweetener calories to be reduced by as much as 80 percent. How do they do that? A one-gram packet of Splenda (3.3 calories) has the power of one-teaspoon of sugar (16.3 calories).

Note- Sweeteners are packaged in tiny packages containing less than 5 calories per packet in order to meet FDA standards for "no-calorie" foods.

Do pay attention to the number of calories in artificial sweetener per the number of calories in the equivalent weight of sugar.

Saccharin (example: Sweet'N Low)

Discovered in 1879, saccharin is the oldest non-nutritional sweetener. World War 1 sugar shortages resulted in more use of saccharin as did

Denise Marks, M.D.

low-calorie food products in the 60's. Unstable when heated, saccharin is not used in bakery products. It is most commonly used in beverages, candy, medications and toothpaste.

Sweet'N Low is primarily composed of saccharin and dextrose.

10 grams contain 9g of dextrose and a calorie count of 36.

10 grams of sugar contains 39 calories.

Aspartame (example: Equal) 200 x sweeter than sugar.

Aspartame comes from amino acids and is used as a table top sweetener. In addition to the small packets for daily use, aspartame is also added to a variety of foods including chewing gum, candy, cereals and soft drinks. Like saccharin, aspartame is not suitable for baking. It actually loses its sweetness when heated.

Note- People with PKU (rare phenylketonuria disorder) cannot metabolize phenylalanine. They should avoid using it or consuming products containing it. Some people complain of headaches and dizziness from aspartame use.

10 grams contain 8g of dextrose, .84 g of starch (Maltodextrin), and aspartame.

The calorie count for 10 grams is 36.

10 grams of sugar contain 39 calories.

Neotame: 8,000 to 13,000 times sweeter than ordinary table sugar. Similar to aspartame, neotame is more stable and has a sweeter taste.

When Neotame is hydrolyzed, part of the result is wood alcohol (methanol). Since neotame is used in tiny amounts, the amount of methanol produced is less than that found in fruit juices. The United

States Food & Drug Administration approved neotame for general use in July of 2002.

Note- aspartic acid is one of the 20 amino acids that make up proteins and about one in 500 of the different amino acid groups in nature.

Acesuflame Potassium (Acesulfame K, Ace K): 200 times sweeter than table sugar.

Found in Coca Cola "Zero." Like saccharin, Ace K in high concentrations has a slightly bitter aftertaste.

Sucralose (example: Splenda) 600 times sweeter than table sugar.

Unlike many other artificial sweeteners, sucralose can be used in cold or hot beverages and in baked goods. It is stable in both cold and hot temperatures. While it is advertised as a no-calorie product, Splenda contains sugars and starch.

10gm contain 9 g of carbohydrates (made of sugars and starch).

The calorie count for 10gm is 33. 10gm of sugar contain 39 calories.

Cyclamate (Sucaryl & Sugar Twin): 30 to 50 times sweeter than sugar. Banned in the United States since 1970 (test rats came down with bladder cancer) Cyclamate still in use in many other countries.

Xylitol: natural sugar alcohol found in fruits and vegetables. Xylitol is not fully utilized by the body and is slowly absorbed. It comes from xylose and contains 40% fewer calories than sugar. Common uses of xylitol include "sugar-free" gum and candy.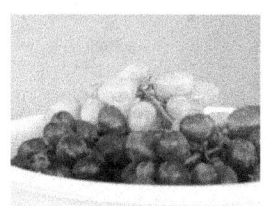

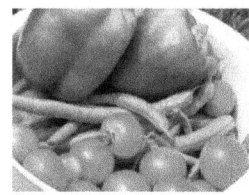 **Sorbitol** (aka glucitol): natural sugar alcohol found in fruits and vegetables. It comes from

21

Denise Marks, M.D.

glucose and is commonly found in "sugar-free" gum and candy.

Erythritol: 60 to 70% as sweet as table sugar.

A natural sugar alcohol found in fruits and vegetables.

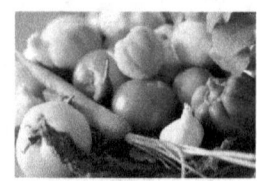

Erythritol is created commercially by fermenting glucose with yeast.

1gm contains 0.2 calories.

There are several other sugar alcohols, including lactitol, maltitol, and mannitol. Sugar alcohols can cause bloating, diarrhea and gas when fermented by micro flora in the gut. As few as 10gm of Sorbitol has been known to cause gastrointestinal problems. Erythritol, on the other hand, does not cause gastric distress. Nor does it promote tooth decay.

Steviol aka Stevia (Truvia, PureVia): Up to 300 times the sweetness of sugar.

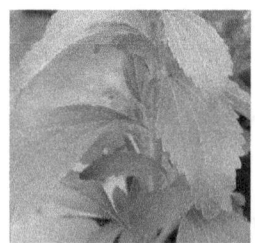

Stevia is the name of a bush. The leaves are the part of the bush processed to create sweeteners.

In the U.S., Stevia is advertised as an herbal supplement rather than as a food additive.

Test results on mammals show high doses of stevioside (one of the ingredients in the leaves) decrease sperm production in males and lead to smaller and fewer offspring in females.

Both Truvia and PureVia contain erythritol as an added ingredient.

3.5gm of Truvia (one packet) contains 3gm of erythritol and un-named natural flavors.

Mogroside V (Nectresse): Approximately 300 times sweeter than sugar.

Extracted from monk fruit (Luo Han Guo), Nectresse has been used in Chinese traditional medicine for about 1000 years. The fruit contains five different mogrosides, all of which account for the sweetness of Nectresse.

Brazzein (Cweet) : About 1000 times sweeter than sugar. Modified corn created Brazzein is up to 1200 times sweeter than sucrose.

A protein extracted from Oubli, the fruit of a West African vine, Brazzein has a taste similar to sucrose. The aftertaste is sweet. Its stability at varying temperatures makes this sweetener practical for many uses.

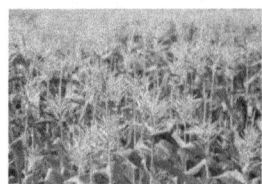

While it isn't usually feasible to try to extract large quantities of Brazzein directly from the fruit, it is possible to produce from corn that has been genetically altered.

Denise Marks, M.D.

CONSUMPTION OF SUGAR

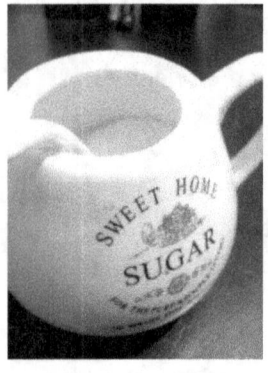 Sugar is a big part of the human diet in most parts of the world. Adding sugar to foods makes the food taste better and provides energy upon consumption. Studies show that an average of 53 pounds of sugar (more than 250 food calories per day) was consumed per individual, worldwide, in 1999. That amount is predicted to rise to 55 pounds per person per year by 2015.

This is quite a contrast to sugar consumption pre-1900 when people averaged only 5 pounds (approximately 30 food calories) per person per year. In the United States, consumption of refined sugar products has ranged from 60 to 100 pounds in the past 40 years. Today, in industrial countries, an estimated average of 100 pounds of sugar (500 calories/day) is eaten per person, per year.

One Pound of Sugar = 454 grams / 1016 calories.
One Cup of Sugar = 774 calories.

When you consider that 16 ounces of most soft drinks contains 160 calories or 10 teaspoons of sugar (as do many fruit juices sold today), it is easy to see how Americans are consuming vast amounts of sugar.

While it's true that sugar provides energy and makes food taste better, it's also true that sugar contains no nutrition value and is the root cause of many modern day diseases, including terminal illnesses.

One teaspoon of sugar contains 3 to 8 grams of sugar depending on the size or fineness of the sugar crystals (powdered sugar being the highest in calories per weight or tsp measurement. That means one teaspoon contains 16 calories to 32 calories. (1 grams = 4 calories of sucrose).

NUTRITIONAL FACTORS INVOLVED IN THE CONSUMPTION OF SUGAR

The average American consumes an astounding 2-3 pounds of sugar each week, which is about 1,000 grams, 4,000 calories and 570 calories per person per day just from the consumption of sugar alone.

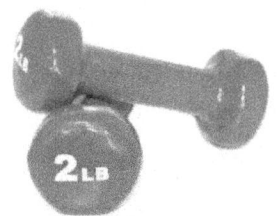

This should not be surprising considering that highly refined sugars in the forms of sucrose (table sugar), dextrose (corn sugar), and high-fructose corn syrup are being processed into so many commonly purchased foods that are consumed daily.

Some of these high glycemic foods include: soft drinks, processed fruit juices, bread, jellies, breakfast cereal, peanut butter, mayonnaise, ketchup, spaghetti sauce, boost and other protein supplements and a plethora of microwavable meals.

Note- Both a 16 oz soft drink and/or 16 oz processed fruit juice contain 40 grams of sugar which is equal to 10 teaspoons of sugar which is equal to 160 calories due to sugar.

Remember - 1 gram of sugar equals four (4) calories so 16 ounces of these processed sweet tasting drinks contain 160 calories (40 grams) due to sugars and one teaspoon of sugar equals 16 calories.

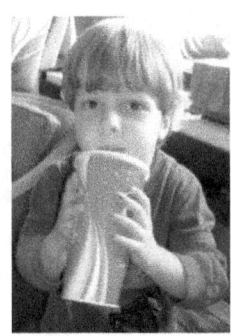

Many people today, especially young people, drink 4 to 5 soft drinks, sweet tea and/or processed fruit juices a day. That adds up to either 640 or 800 calories a day coming from sugar alone.

Then taking these daily 640 or 800 calories times 7, you can get 4,480 to 5,600 calories or

Denise Marks, M.D.

1,120 to 1,400 grams of sugar a week. Then divide these weekly gram numbers by 454 grams it is easy to see how the researchers arrived at the 2 to 3 pounds of sugar a week per person. Is this, 2 to 3 pounds of sugar a week, not overwhelming!

Now consider how much sugar is consumed per the average person in one year.

Prior to the turn of this century (1887-1890), the average consumption was only 5 to 10 lbs. (approximately 2,350 to 4,700 grams or 9,400 18,800 calories) per person per year!

In the last 20 years, we have increased sugar consumption in the U.S. from 24 pounds to 100 to 150 lbs. of sugar per person per year! That is an increase from 10,000 to now 45,400 to 68,000 grams of sugar per year!

Remember from high school math, one (1) pound contains 454 grams and 454 grams times 4 (the number of calories in one gram of sugar) equals 1,816 calories! This means we Americans are consuming between 181,600 calories to 272,000 calories a year from sugar -just from sugar. And the really bad news is that sugar contains no good nutritious nutrients.

Recommended Daily Consumption of Sugar by the American Heart Association

Sugar intake must be monitored in a healthy diet though some sugar is necessary for good health. Without knowing what constitutes a healthy sugar intake, you can easily exceed the recommended limit because sugar is included in many foods, regardless of whether they are sweet or savory. Health care agencies such as the American Heart Association provide guidelines on recommended intakes for sugar.

Note- Recommended sugar intake refers to added sugar. This means that daily intake guidelines do not apply to certain foods such as fruits, which are natural sources of sugar. These fruit sugars do not pose as much of a risk to your diet.

The problem with sugar occurs when it is added to foods and beverages. These foods include coffee, tea, soda, desserts and even condiments and sauces such as ketchup and mayonnaise. Sugar is often added to products in the form of corn syrup, honey, sorghum, maple syrup, high fructose corn syrup, dextrose and sucrose as well as sweeteners. You should always look at ingredient labels of products for these added sugars.

Recommended Grams of Sugar for Men: As caloric and nutritional intakes vary between men and women, so do recommendations for sugar in grams. The American Heart Association states that men should not consume more than 45 grams of sugar in a day.

Recommended Grams of Sugar for Women: The recommended sugar intake for women is less than that of men. The AHA advises women to limit their intake of sugar to 30 grams of sugar each day.

The recommended daily calorie consumption varies from 1,500 calories for people doing desk work to 2,800 calories for those doing moderate heavy work. And only 30 grams or 120 calories of sugar a day for women and 45 grams or 180 calories of sugar a day for men is recommended. This is possible when one sets their minds to eating foods that are not high glycemic or have the added sugar in them during preparing or processing.

Today, more than ever, there are more and more questions and studies on the role of individual sugars and sugar substitutes on human health and medical diseases, especially refined sugars such as high fructose corn syrup.

Denise Marks, M.D.

Blood glucose levels

Professionals once believed that sugar raised blood glucose levels faster than starch because sugar is chemically simpler. This belief has been proven wrong. There is no longer a reason to look at sugar or starch individually when seeking to control blood glucose levels in those suffering from diabetes.

Carbohydrate counting is now the method used to plan diabetic meals. While sugar and starch affect blood glucose levels the same, they differ when it comes to oral health. Sugar is more likely to cause cavities.

CONVERSION TABLE FOR SUCROSE THE MOST COMMON SIMPLE SUGAR

Dry Goods - Sugar Conversion table for converting cups to grams to ounces

Note- 454g equal 1 lb (one pound) equal 16 oz and 454g equal one (1) pound

One tsp equal 5g and one Tablespoon equal 15g equal 60 calories of sugar

One Tablespoon equal 3 tsp

2 Tablespoons equal 1/8 cup or 16g or 563 oz

1/4 cup 32 g 1.13 oz

1/2 cup 64 g 2.25 oz

1 cup   128 g 4.5 oz = ¼ lb or(4 cups equal 1 pound)

SUGAR METABOLISM

Carbohydrates contain sugar your body metabolizes into energy. Carbs also affect substances in the brain that can impact appetite, mood and sleep.

Glucose is the sugar that the cells utilize for energy. When your body absorbs glucose, it stimulates insulin secretion into the blood stream. Insulin is a hormone that carries glucose from your blood into your cells. Insulin also manages the movement of amino acids from your blood into your skeletal muscle cells.

It is interesting to note that increasing your consumption of complex or simple sugars results in increased production of neurotransmitters in the brain.

FRUCTOSE METABOLISM

High-fructose corn syrup (HFCS) is a refined form of sugar. Since it has been refined from its original form, the body metabolizes it differently than the glucose form. When you consume HFCS, it is up to your liver to metabolize it.

1. Fructose elevates uric acid. Elevated uric acid then decreases nitric oxide. This raises the hormone angiotension, causing smooth muscle cells to contract. The contraction raises your blood pressure and puts your kidneys at risk of being damaged.

2. Fructose is known to chronically inflame blood vessels, which leads to weakening of the lining of arteries. The LDL (La)-cholesterol becomes magnetized to the inflamed area and gets imbedded into the lining of the artery causing blockage of that artery. This blockage is responsible for causing hypertension, heart attacks and strokes.

Denise Marks, M.D.

3. Also, a good deal of evidence exists that some cancers are caused by the chronic inflammation that is due to excess of both fructose and glucose in the blood stream. However, it is mainly the higher percentage of fructose to glucose from high fructose corn syrup that instigates these changes.

4. NOTE- CANCER, CARDIOVASCULAR DISEASE AND NEURO-PSYCH METABOLIC DISEASES (DEMENTIA, ALZHEIMER, DEPRESSION, ANXIETY)- were virtually unknown before HIGH FRUCTOSE CORN SYRUP as a low cost "sugar" became popular in the mid 1900's.

HIGH FRUCTOSE CORN SYRUP - FRUCTOSE - TRICKS YOUR BRAIN AND YOUR BODY

High Fructose Corn Syrup tricks your mind and your body in many ways. The most significant and acute (not chronic) way is in the way high fructose corn syrup fools your metabolism.

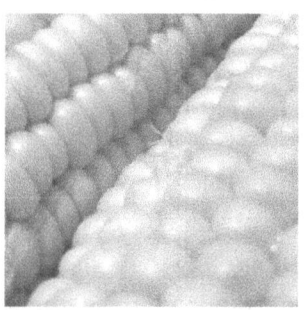

High Fructose Corn Syrup actually turns off your body's appetite-control system!

High Fructose Corn Syrup does not appropriately stimulate insulin (the hormone that is responsible for transporting glucose into every cell for energy production). High Fructose Corn Syrup does not suppress, but stimulates ghrelin (the "hunger hormone ") so you stay hungry -longer: and (HFCS) does not stimulate leptin, the "satiety hormone", so you stay even hungrier longer.

Together, the increase in ghrelin and the reduction of leptin's satiety effect result in you eating much more than you would if HFCS was not in the foods you consumed. And of course this altered metabolism and the effect of suppressing ghrelin and reducing leptin's satiety effect is what leads to weight gain.

And for some unexplained reason this combination of high fructose corn syrup and the hormone imbalances it creates in the body - leads especially to abdominal obesity "beer belly".

Fructose also plays a significant role in the development of insulin resistance and all the metabolic diseases that are a part of the metabolic syndrome that is connected to insulin resistance. High fructose corn syrup causes this damage by first, stimulating a decrease in the good HDL-cholesterol and stimulating an increase in the bad LDL-cholesterol as well as elevating triglycerides, elevating blood sugar, which increases blood pressure—i.e., the classics symptoms of the metabolic syndrome.

The metabolism of high fructose corn syrup is very similar to the metabolism of ethanol (alcohol). Both of these chemical have a multitude of toxic (damaging) effects on cells, tissues and organs of the body, but especially on the liver. In the liver, where fructose is metabolized, the damage done by the overload of metabolizing excess fructose is known to cause non-alcoholic fatty liver disease.

High Fructose Corn Syrup is also known as "alcohol without the buzz". These changes are not seen when humans or animals eat non-refined starch and/or glucose, suggesting that high fructose corn syrup is a "bad carbohydrate" especially when fructose of any kind is consumed in excess of 25 grams (100 calories) per day.

EATING "HIGH FRUCTOSE CORN SYRUP" IS FAR WORSE THAN EATING "FAT"

This concept of HFCS verses fat causing most of our modern metabolic medical diseases, especially heart disease and diabetes, has been debated by scientists and nutritionalists alike for more than 40 years.

Denise Marks, M.D.

There are two overall reasons high fructose corn syrup is worse than fat in causing internal damaged to cell receptors and causes imbalances of hormones:

(1) People are consuming fructose in enormous quantities, which has made the negative effects much more profound. The massive consumption of HFCS containing sodas is the major cause of the explosion of our modern day metabolic medical diseases.

(2) Today, 55 percent of sweeteners used in beverages and manufactured processed foods come from high fructose corn syrup. The number one source of empty non-nutritive calories in America is - soda beverages that contain high fructose corn syrup.

Food and beverage manufacturers began switching their sweeteners from sucrose to high fructose corn syrup in the 1970s when they discovered that HFCS was not only far cheaper to make, but is also about 20 percent sweeter than conventional table sugar - sucrose.

SUMMARY OF HIGH FRUCTOSE CORN SYRUP

It is well known that excess high fructose corn syrup in the blood stream causes health issues:

1 HFCS contains the same two sugars as sucrose but in a more harmful percentage of fructose metabolically speaking due to its chemical structure.

2. The fructose and the glucose are not bound together in HFCS, as they are in table sugar, so your body doesn't have to break it down. Therefore, the higher percentage of fructose is absorbed immediately, going straight to your liver. There are some major differences in how different sugars are broken down and used by the human body.

3. After eating fructose, most of the metabolic burden rests on your liver. This is NOT the case with glucose, of which your liver breaks down only 20 percent.

4. Nearly every cell in your body utilizes glucose for energy, so it's normally "burned up- used up" faster after consumption: whereas fructose is not used immediately for energy. It has to go through enzymatic (chemical) changes in the liver that have to convert fructose to glucose.

5. Any excess of fructose from high fructose corn syrup in the blood stream, immediately gets turned into FAT (VLDL and triglycerides), which means more fat deposits accumulate throughout your body but especially around the middle.

6. HFCS causes erectile dysfunction by decreasing the amount of nitric acid in the blood stream. (Viagra and Cialis increase nitric acid and so does eating watermelon and figs).

7. HFCS triggers high blood pressure by increasing angiotension.

8. Fructose actually turns off your body's appetite-control system causing one to always feel hungry. Fructose from high fructose corn syrup does not suppress ghrelin (the "hunger hormone ") so you remain hungry. Also, it doesn't stimulate leptin (the "satiety hormone"), which decreasing the effect of these two hormones together result in you eating more than normal: which then leads to weight gain and abdominal obesity ("beer belly").

9. Fructose from high fructose corn syrup does not appropriately stimulate insulin.

10. Fructose from high fructose corn syrup also plays a significant role in the development of insulin resistance and leptin resistance. Insulin resistance (IR) is now known to be the root of the problem when it comes to all the metabolic diseases that are a part of the metabolic

33

syndrome. It does this by decreasing HDL, increasing LDL, elevating triglycerides, elevating blood sugar, and high blood pressure—i.e., the classic metabolic syndrome.

11. Fructose metabolism is very similar to ethanol metabolism, which has a multitude of toxic (damaging) effects, including NAFLD (non-alcoholic fatty liver disease). It's alcohol without the buzz.

Your body metabolizes high fructose corn syrup much differently than it metabolizes glucose. The entire burden of metabolizing high fructose corn syrup or fructose from any source, falls directly on your liver, and when there is excess fructose in the blood stream, due to the consumption of high fructose corn syrup containing food and sodas, it is quickly converted into fat and stored first in the liver and then in the adipose cells of the body.

 This explanation of the metabolism of fructose explains not only weight gain and the obesity connection, but also abdominal obesity (beer belly).

Abdominal obesity is much more noticeable today in so many Americans than it was before 1970 when the explosion of processed food and drinks containing high fructose corn syrup occurred.

High Fructose Corn Syrup is known to be:

(1) the primary cause of non-alcoholic fatty liver.

(2) the primary cause of most kidney diseases.

 (3) the leading cause of chronic inflammation. Note- chronic inflammation is at the core of most chronic metabolic, deadly, medical diseases."

Also, High Fructose Corn Syrup is known to:

 (4) trigger weight gain (obesity),

(5) trigger the production of cholesterol and triglycerides - causing heart disease,

(6) trigger insulin resistance - causing diabetes,

(7) causes arthritis and other inflammatory diseases by increases uric acid through a complex process that causes cells to burn up their ATP rapidly, leading to "cell shock" and increased cell death.

Note- After eating excessive amounts of high fructose corn syrup, cells become starved of energy, that has to come from glucose or ketone bodies, and then these cells enter a state of shock, just as if they have lost their blood supply.

(8) High fructose corn syrup feeds cancer cells. It does this- by triggering the production of ribose sugar, the raw material of DNA. Note- It's easier for cancer cells to make ribose (for DNA) from fructose than it is for cancer cells to make ribose for DNA from any other source.

However, if you do consume tiny amounts of high fructose corn syrup, you don't necessarily trigger the massive production of ribose in cancer cells. Eating no more than about 15 grams (3 teaspoons) twice a day won't trigger the nasty reactions that accelerate cancer proliferation and other metabolic medical diseases.

CHECKING LABELS

When evaluating carbs, look at both the fiber content — it should be high — and the glycemic index (the sugar/fiber ratio) which should be low.

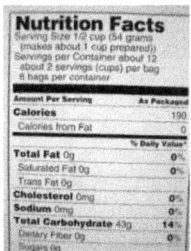

Note- The words "whole grain" on a package can often be misleading. Remember to determine this value use the 10 to 1 rule. Look for a ratio of 10

Denise Marks, M.D.

grams of carbs to 1 gram of fiber to determine whether the product is truly whole grain.

For example: If the bread label has 40 grams of carbs per serving and 4 grams of fiber, the ratio is 10 to 1 - which is good. If it the bread label has 40 grams of carbs and 2 grams of fiber, its carb/fiber ratio is 20 to 1 which is not so good.

Note also, all processed "**low fat**" food will <u>always</u> contain added sugar and/or salt. **Just check the labels!** The FDA has required that the food industry accurately label all ingredients that are in a given serving.

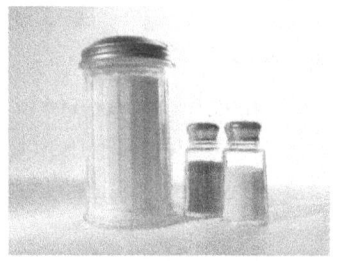

They are required to list the <u>most abundant ingredient first</u> and <u>end with the least abundant</u> ingredient. They are also required to list the percentage of fat, protein, sugar, fiber, cholesterol, salt (sodium) and calories per serving.

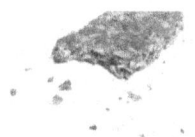

In a popular online illustration, comparisons were made between breakfast bars and cupcakes. The breakfast bar (Quaker Oats brand) had a sugar/fiber ratio of 6, a little bit higher than the recommended norm. The carb/fiber ratio of the bar was around 14, higher than the recommended rule.

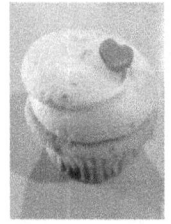

The cupcake, however, was the worst dietary culprit – it had a sugar/fiber ratio of 36! (18gm of sugar divided by .o5 gm of fiber.) The carb/fiber ratio was no better. (26 divided by.05 =53!)

While you may find these examples extreme, they are not. Processed foods contain sugar to make up for the "low fat" content. Real sugar is removed. It is then replaced with artificial sweeteners or trans-fats.

Food processing companies continue to add sugar to everything to balance out the low fat content. Food companies either 1) take out fat and replace it with real sugar or artificial sweeteners or 2) remove all of the real sugar and replace it with trans-fat products or artificial sweeteners.

Natural sugar is found in all carbohydrates. In unprocessed natural carbohydrates, fiber is added with the sugar.

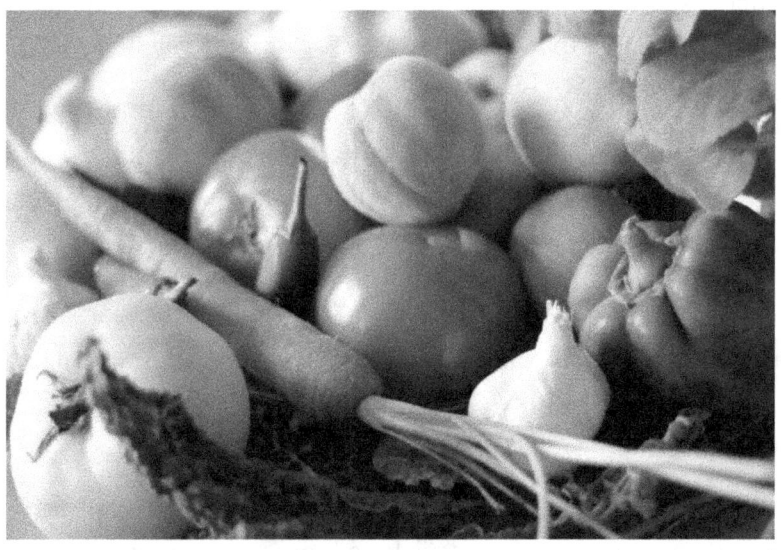

Examples include fruits, vegetables, nuts and grains.

Denise Marks, M.D.

RECOMMENDED PERCENTAGE OF SUGAR THAT MAY STILL BE "OK"

Given the vast variety of food types, it's not always possible to calculate the percentage of certain nutrients, especially in many of the processed foods when they contain artificial sweeteners. Instead of focusing on just the percentage of sugar these carbohydrate foods contain, it is better to consider the positive nutritional aspects of the food, such as the total fiber content and micronutrients in that food.

This is true whether it is fruit, vegetables, whole grain products, lean protein and/or processed foods that contain sugar as well as the type and amount of fats that food contains. Note- if the food contains artificial sweeteners it really becomes difficult to calculate the sugar/fiber ratio. That is because these artificial sweeteners affect the metabolism of those foods differently.

The important issue to remember is that by avoiding products with added sugars, you'll be consuming a product that's more nutritionally dense. Note again: 100 calories of unsugared strawberries provide more healthy nutrients than 100 calories of sugar sweetened strawberries. Therefore, the unsweetened strawberries are said to be more nutritionally dense. Another way of saying this is unsugared strawberries contain more fiber and healthy nutrients per calorie than the sugar sweetened strawberries.

It can be very difficult to estimate the portion of calories coming from added sugars for processed grain based carbohydrate products, such as cereals, granola bars, breads, etc., as well as processed foods that contain high fructose corn syrup or nonnutritive, artificial sweeteners.

However, you can make a reasonable estimate of the "wholeness" of grain cereals or grain breads by using the carb/fiber ratio and the carb/sugar ratio. Remember, to calculate the carb/fiber ratio of a cereal that has 40 grams of carbohydrates and 5 grams of fiber- simply divide the total grams of carbohydrates in that (stated) serving by the number of grams of fiber in that serving. The carb/fiber ratio is 8 which means there are 8 grams of carbs to 1 gram of fiber. **This numerical value "8" is considered a low and healthy carb/fiber ratio**.

Now consider the carb/sugar ratio. If the carbohydrate value is 40g and the sugar content per serving is 30g. Then the carb/sugar ratio is 40g divided by 30g which equals 1.3. This means there is 1.3 grams of carbohydrates for every 1 gram of sugar.

 This time when the numerically value is low it is a bad sign as it means most of the carbohydrate is pure sugar which also means that this food contains very little whole grain. It would be a healthier cereal if the carbohydrate value was 40g and the sugar value was 5g.

The carb/sugar ratio would be 40g divided by 5g which is 8. When using the carb/sugar ratio to determine the nutritional value of a food then a higher number is better. A high carb/sugar ratio means there is more whole grains and less added sugars.

Note- The carb/sugar ratios and the carb/fiber ratios are not the same as the sugar/fiber ratio. And it is the sugar/fiber ratio that determines the glycemic value of carbohydrate containing food. The glycemic value of food is closer in value to the sugar/fiber ratio.

And a low glycemic value as well as a low sugar/fiber ratio is healthier than a high glycemic value or high sugar/fiber ratio. Remember, lower numbers are better when it comes to the glycemic value as well as the sugar/fiber ratio and the carb/fiber ratio.

Also Note- foods that contain high carb/fiber ratios tend to be indicative of foods that contain very little whole grains and lots of sugar or enriched refined flour. When the amount of fiber is low and the amount of sugar or carbohydrates is high - then the sugar/fiber

Denise Marks, M.D.

ratio or the carb/fiber ratio will be high as well as the glycemic value will be high and the nutritional value of that food is low.

Another way of stating this concept is - the higher the amount of fiber per carb or fiber per sugar means - that food contains more whole grains and fiber and less added sugar. Therefore these foods would be more nutritional. It has already been determined by many nutritionists that a <u>healthy cereal or bread</u> product will have a carb/fiber ratio of less than 10. Note- an even better way to base a healthy percentage of carbs is to calculate the sugar/fiber ratio which should be 4 or less.

THE EFFECT OF SUGAR ON APPETITE

Simple sugars occur naturally in fruits, vegetables and grains. These natural foods are nutritious staples in any healthy diet because they contain lots of fiber. The simple sugars you need to be aware of and on the lookout for are added simple sugars.   In addition to the damage they inflict on the body, simple sugars that contain no fiber actually promote hunger, causing dieters to eat even more. The more you eat, the more at risk you are for gaining weight.

Most people, however, don't pay attention to the effect that sugar may have on their appetite. **They just know they're never quite satisfied after a sweet tasting, sugar laden drink or breakfast and are usually looking for unhealthier foods not long after having these high sugar / low fiber breakfast foods or liquids**. The reason for this dilemma is - that processed foods which are high in sugar and low in fiber are also considered <u>high glycemic</u> carbohydrates. These foods are absorbed quickly and thus raise the insulin level higher and quicker than normal which then alters the metabolism of any high glycemic carbohydrate, especially those that contain high fructose corn syrup and/or artificial sweeteners.

Remember: the consumption of simple sugars without the necessary fiber - causes a spike in blood sugar and thus a spike in blood insulin levels. **This surge in insulin is then followed by a crash in ones level of blood sugar**. This severe sudden decrease in the blood sugar can cause symptoms of **hypoglycemia**, e.g., anxiety disorders, attention deficit disorders (ADD), headaches, dizziness, slurred speech and even seizures. Also, this drop in blood sugar leaves one feeling even hungrier than they were before they consumed these high glycemic products- and more likely they will continue to eat until they can find something that will satisfy and make them feel "full".

If you've ever consumed something like a 16 ounce cola drink or a candy bar in place of lunch on a busy day, you may have experienced any of the symptoms of hypoglycemia mentioned above or you may have had the feeling of "I need to eat something more- quickly". You may also experience the feeling of not being satisfied. Perhaps you have had a doughnut every morning on the way to work yet still find yourself looking for the vending machines not long after you arrive.

Whatever your sugar vice, the effects are - for the most part - the same: which is, it leaves you feeling more hungry and less satisfied. These symptoms of hypoglycemia are basically due to the surge of insulin that was release in response to the high amount of sugar (glucose) that was rapidly absorbed into the blood stream.

Note. Insulin is known as the hunger hormone, the fat storage hormone and the weight causing hormone. When your insulin level is high, you will most likely give in to your hunger, and then you will eat more calories than you can actually burn as energy, and before you know it, you're up a notch on your belt buckle or you may receive a bad diagnosis of one or more of the many modern-day, inflammatory, metabolic diseases from your doctor.

Note- Dr. Oz reminds people to look at how many total grams of sugar are in a serving of that product as well as the total grams of

fiber that product has per serving. You can then divide the sugar grams by the fiber grams in order to get the sugar/fiber ratio which should be less than 3 or 4. This information is a powerful tool in assessing the glycemic value, health or nutritional value of your food choices.

Remember: The simplest and most useful marker that determines the nutritional value of foods that contain carbohydrates is - the "sugar/fiber" ratio. This ratio is technically different than the carb/fiber ratio that is often calculated and reported instead of the sugar/fiber ratio. And it is the amount of fiber per sugar in these carbohydrates basically determines the glycemic value or nutritional value of that food. Also remember that a low glycemic choice is healthier than a high glycemic choice.

A healthy, low glycemic food has about a 3 to 1 sugar/fiber ratio or lower. For example, a 1 to 1 sugar/fiber ratio means that if the sugar content is 5 or 8 then the fiber content also has to be 5 or 8 respectively: and a 1 to 2 sugar/fiber ratio means the sugar content is only one half of a gram for every 1 gram of fiber: and a 1 to 6 sugar/fiber ratio, (the best ratio in this discussion), means the sugar content is only one sixth of a gram for every 1 gram of fiber. Another way of explaining this value 1 to 6 sugar/fiber ratio would be if the product contained 10 grams of sugar and 60 grams of fiber: or the product contained 5 grams of sugar and 30 grams of fiber.

Ironically and sadly, the current U.S. average sugar/fiber ratio is about a 12 to 1 or simply 12. This is the result of the food industry adding sugar to just about all manufactured or processed foods as well as the removal of fiber and other natural nutrients during the processing of "low fat" unhealthy foods. Removing good fiber and adding sugar is done by the food industry in order to not only add a longer shelf life to that product but also to make the "low fat" foods taste better and to decrease the satiety value of that food products. All of these reasons will cause you to want to <u>eat more and more</u> of sweet tasting, low fat foods in an attempt to become satisfied.

To get a healthy 3 to 1 sugar/fiber ratio during a 24 hour period of time and still get the natural fiber content to be the recommended 30 grams of fiber, the total sugar would be 90 grams or <u>360 calories</u> coming from sugar (90 divided by 30 equals the 3 to 1 ratio). A 24 hour diet with an even better sugar/fiber ratio of 1 to 1 and still get the 30 grams of fiber would contain only 30 grams of sugar or 120 calories of sugar which is about <u>one</u> small cola drink or 8 ounces of a processed apple or orange juice drink. Remember that <u>200 calories</u> (50 grams) a day coming from sugar is the 'total' recommended daily amount of sugar for a 24 hour period of time.

Sadly, the average daily (24 hour) intake of fiber in the U.S. population today - is about 12-15 grams, while the average sugar intake is 200 to 300 grams (or about 800 to 1,200 calories from sugar alone). This sugar/fiber ratio would be 300 divided by 15 which equals 20 to 1 and can also be stated as "<u>20</u>". <u>Note- This 300 grams of sugar (1,200 calories or the equivalent of 6 glasses of coke products) is the amount of sugar added daily in most American diets: and not the 50 grams (200 calories) as recommended.</u>

It is no secret that sodas (carbonated beverages-coke, Pepsi, etc.) are an important part of American culture. Soda machines are found everywhere from out front at convenience stores to the back room of factories and businesses.

The sugary beverages may be in high demand but they're also high in sugar calories while containing absolutely no healthy ingredients. According to the Coca-Cola website, a 12 oz can of regular coke contains 40gm of sugar (160 calories.) A 16 oz serving of the drink contains about 50gm of sugar (200 calories).

Coca Cola contains nothing of dietary value. There's no fiber, fat or protein in it. The ingredients list reveals: carbonated water sweetened with high fructose corn syrup, caramel color, phosphoric acid, natural flavors and caffeine. Truly a recipe for disaster when it comes to diet.

One cup of sugar = 200gm (800 calories.) Can you imagine picking up a spoon and eating a full cup of sugar daily? That's what many young Americans do every day.

one 12 oz high fructose corn syrup drink (cola as well as processed juices and sweet tea) contains 40 grams of sugar. And this amount of sugar is equal to 10 teaspoons of table sugar (one teaspoon of sugar equals 4 grams which equals 16 calories: so 10 teaspoons would equal 160 calories (10 x 16).

THE VALUE OF EATING WHOLE GRAINS!

Why bother eating whole grains? The answer is because they deliver everything that an intact whole grain has to offer, i.e., fiber, germ, bran, vitamins, minerals, antioxidants, and one or more specific phytonutrients.

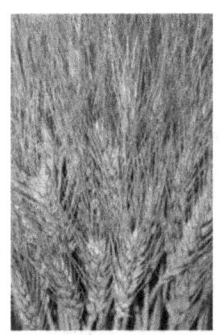

As long as the whole grains aren't over-processed, over-heated, over-refined, the body digests these whole grain foods more slowly, which can provide more satiety (satisfaction) and delay the hunger feeling.

 Some long-term studies have shown that consuming whole grains (more fiber - less simple carbohydrates) is one way to help reduce the odds of developing heart disease, diabetes, and other chronic, modern-day, inflammatory, metabolic medical conditions. Not only are whole grain products healthier they often taste better than processed grains.

Note again, the body digests the whole grain foods more slowly, and therefore whole grain foods provide more satiety (satisfaction) and delay the hunger feeling.

Intact whole grains, e.g., wheat berries, oat berries, brown rice, quinoa, and the like,—are the best source of whole grains. Ground whole grains come next, as long as they still deliver a good dose of fiber and as long as there is no added sugar, trans-fats, or sodium. To find the healthy whole grain products, use the 10:1 carb/fiber guide mentioned above.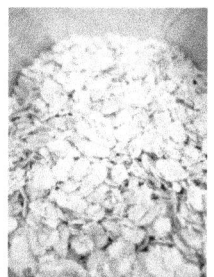

SUGAR IS THE ACTUAL "DRIVING FORCE" THAT TRIGGERS OR CAUSES MOST OF OUR MODERN DAY METABOLIC, INFLAMMATORY, MEDICAL DISEASES

Again, some examples of these modern-day, inflammatory, metabolic, medical diseases are: **diabetes, obesity, hypercholesterolemia, hypertriglyceridemia, hypertension, heart disease, kidney and eye diseases, arthritis, most neurological and psychological diseases and even many cancers, etc**.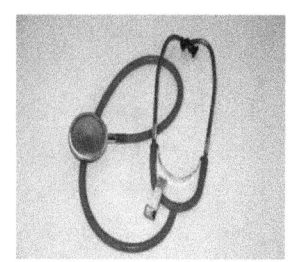

These inflammatory metabolic diseases have been further classified under the general heading of "the Metabolic Syndrome". And inflammation at the cellular level has been identified as the actual cause of these diseases that are considered as diseases of the Metabolic Syndrome.

Denise Marks, M.D.

Diseases due to inflammation are caused by both the chronic high levels of blood sugar (glucose) and higher than normal levels of insulin as well as toxins and free radicals. These two chemicals (sugar and insulin) can actually cause internal inflammatory damage within blood vessels, nerves, cell membranes as well as many receptors on the cell membranes. The other culprit that is at the root of these modern-day inflammatory metabolic medical diseases is oxidative stress and free radicals.

Oxidative stress has been linked to not only inflammation in general but also to heart disease, Alzheimer's disease and a host of other modern-day, inflammatory, metabolic, medical diseases. Inflammation can also be caused by the production of free radicals, which damage DNA and alter the structure of key proteins.

Damage due to oxidative stress is damage to cells caused by an excess of free radicals. **In a process similar to rusting of metal**, the rogue free radicals damage DNA and inhibit cellular metabolism & energy generation. (*Free radicals will be discussed later*).

It is well known that the excessive consumption of sugars has been linked with most modern-day, metabolic diseases, abnormalities and/or adverse health conditions.

 This is not only because excessive consumption of sugars causes a shortage of the essential nutrients to be consumed, but also because high concentrations of sugar in the blood stream can cause damaged receptors. These damaged receptors cause what is known as Insulin Resistance. And Insulin Resistance is also known as Type 2 Diabetes Mellitus (DM).

Note- A large percentage of popular cereals on our grocery store shelves contain massive amounts of sugars.

Sugars (simple carbohydrates) are

digested quickly and are usually void of essential micronutrients such as phytonutrients, vitamins, minerals and fiber. You may even be surprised to learn that many cereals advertized as "healthy" cereals are loaded with added sugars.

The majority of sugar sweetened cereals contain at least 15 to 30 grams of sugar or 60 to 120 calories due to sugar alone. This is 4 to 8 teaspoons of table sugar per serving not including what you may add to that cereal. One teaspoon of table sugar equals 4 grams: so, 8 teaspoons equals 32 grams of sugar which equals 128 calories (32 grams x 4 calories) from sugar alone.

The American Heart Association was one of the first to issue formal guidelines on sugar intake. They recommended no more than 100 calories per day, or about 6 teaspoons of sugar for women and no more than 150 calories per day, or about 9 teaspoons of sugar a day for men.

There are many processed food products that are misrepresented to the public as healthy "low fat" -fiber containing foods: when in actuality they are low in fiber and high in sugar. A high sugar to fiber ratio artificially manipulated in modern-day processed food gets or drives people to consume more of these foods and therefore they will buy more of the "taste good", "comfort tasting" foods.

We all should ask ourselves this question: Is the FDA really looking out for the consumer or is it looking out for the food industry?

SUGAR CAUSES MANY OF OUR MODERN DAY DISEASES

Death by sugar is a very profound statement but not an overstatement of the truth.

 The fact is that - sugar is the root cause of nearly all of the metabolic medical diseases that are chronic, and disabling and/or lead to an - early death!

 Scientific evidence is mounting that indicate sugars (especially granulated sugar, sucrose, and high fructose corn syrup, fructose and many starches that break down to simple sugars) are the major agents causing many of today's terminally ill (deadly) metabolic medical diseases. These metabolic diseases are now known to shorten one's life and therefore cause an early death that is actually preventable.

 Note- **metabolic medical diseases** - refer to those medical diseases that are caused by an excess or sugar and insulin in particular and/or a deficiency of certain nutrient(s), enzyme(s) and/or hormone(s), etc.

Some examples of these metabolic medical diseases caused by sugar are listed below both by systems and then by disorders

METABOLIC MEDICAL DISEASE CAUSED BY SUGAR ARE:

Cardiology (Cardiovascular system - Heart and Blood Vessels)

   ischemic heart disease: i.e., angina and myocardial infarction

   congestive heart failure   high blood pressure

   abnormally high cholesterol and triglyceride levels

deep vein thrombosis and pulmonary embolism (a pro-thrombotic state)

Endocrinology and Reproductive systems (Consists of Glands and Hormones)

diabetes mellitus   infertility

polycystic ovarian syndrome   birth defects

menstrual disorders

complications during pregnancy   intrauterine fetal death

Immune System (Consists of Lymph nodes and lymph vessels, Bone marrow-especially WBCs, Spleen and Thymus)

- ✓ Weakened immune system, i.e., immune deficiencies allow infections and cancer to become deadly

- ✓ Overactive immune system allows allergic rhinitis, asthma that can become deadly

- ✓ Auto-immune disorders, i.e., type 1 diabetes, rheumatoid arthritis and lupus can become deadly

Gastrointestinal system (Consists of Organs, Hormones and Enzymes associated with the digestion and metabolism of food)

Gastro-esophageal reflux disease   fatty liver disease

cholelithiasis (gallstones)   colitis and bowel obstruction

irritable bowel syndrome

Denise Marks, M.D.

Neurology (neurological system) Consists of the brain, nerves, hormones)

- stroke
- migraines
- carpal tunnel syndrome
- multiple sclerosis (MS)
- dementia and possibly Alzheimer's Disease
- idiopathic intracranial hypertension

Oncology (Cancers, consisting of a multisystem disorders that usually deals with damaged DNA within each cell)

breast and ovarian cancer

esophageal and colorectal cancers

liver and pancreatic cancers

gallbladder and stomach cancers

endometrial and cervical cancers

prostate and kidney cancers

non-Hodgkin's lymphoma and multiple myeloma

Respirology system (Consists mainly of the lungs and histamines)

obstructive sleep apnea or the obesity hypoventilation syndrome

asthma

increased complications during general anesthesia

Rheumatology and Orthopedics (Consists of the muscle, bones, ligaments and tendons)

gout   poor mobility   osteoarthritis

low back pain   fibromyalgia

Urology and Nephrology (Renal system, i.e., kidneys, bladder, electrolytes and hormones)

erectile dysfunction

urinary incontinence

chronic renal failure

Psychiatry (Deals with the emotional aspect and is the biggest cause of suicide)

> ➢ depression

> ➢ social stigmatization mainly due to overweight issues caused by sugar

Denise Marks, M.D.

A LIST OF SPECIFIC, PREVENTABLE SUGAR-FUELED MEDICAL DISORDERS THAT CAN CAUSE AN EARLY DEATH

Sugar can suppress the immune system and **thus** contribute to a weakened defense against bacterial infections and/or even some cancers.

Sugar can cause free radical formation in the bloodstream which can trigger or cause inflammatory damage of the DNA within each body cell that then leads to the development or growth of many cancers.

Sugar can trigger or cause weight gain and/or obesity by causing hormonal imbalances.

Sugar can increase kidney size and produce pathological (damaging) changes in the kidney that can increase fluid retention in the body and high blood pressure.

Sugar can also increase systolic blood pressure (hypertension) by causing a significant rise in triglycerides and total cholesterol.

Sugar can promote an elevation of harmful or "bad" cholesterol (LDLs) as well as reduce the "good" high density cholesterol (HDLs).

Sugar can increase the risk of coronary heart disease, by causing atherosclerosis, i.e., cardiovascular disease

Sugar can overstress the pancreas, causing damage to the beta cells which leads to decreased glucose tolerance, a decrease in insulin sensitivity, hyperglycemia, and an increased fasting level of blood glucose, i.e., diabetes.

Sugar can cause liver cells to divide, increasing the size of the liver and thus sugar can increase the amount of fat in the liver (fatty liver disease).

Sugar can upset the body's mineral balance, i.e. chromium deficiency and copper deficiency, interferes with absorption of calcium and magnesium.

Sugar: can increases the risk of Crohn's disease, Ulcerative colitis, as well as Celiac disease, producing an acidic stomach and trigger or cause GERD.

Sugar increases bacterial fermentation in the colon causing IBS (irritable bowel syndrome) causing bloating, pain and nutritional deficiencies.

Sugar can cause depression and can cause drowsiness and decreased activity in children as well as hyperactivity, triggering ADHD, (concentration difficulties), anxiety, and crankiness in children and <u>suicide</u> in adults.

Sugar can speed up wrinkles and grey hair and speed up the aging process in general.

Sugar can promote tooth decay and periodontal disease and cause septicemia or bacteremia and even meningitis a very deadly infection.

Sugar can increase blood platelet adhesiveness which increases risk of blood clots (pro-thrombotic state) and cardio-vascular diseases.

Sugar is detrimental to the body. It contains **NO** minerals, **NO** vitamins and **NO** fiber. It has **NOTHING** to offer the body. It negatively affects all of the cells in the body but is known to be particularly harsh on the cells that make up the immune, cardiac, hormone and neurological systems.

Denise Marks, M.D.

Sugar's affect on American diets is well documented. Some researchers suggest that sugar in the diet is one of the 3 most common causes of the deadly (chronic and/or terminal) metabolic medical diseases and the number one cause of obesity. Obesity in and of itself can cause an early death.

GLYCEMIC INDEX OR VALUES

Carbohydrates that are slowly absorbed are called "low glycemic" carbohydrates, while quickly absorbed carbohydrates are called "high glycemic" carbohydrates. The picture below follows two separate blood sugar curves. One following a high glycemic meal and one following a low glycemic meal.

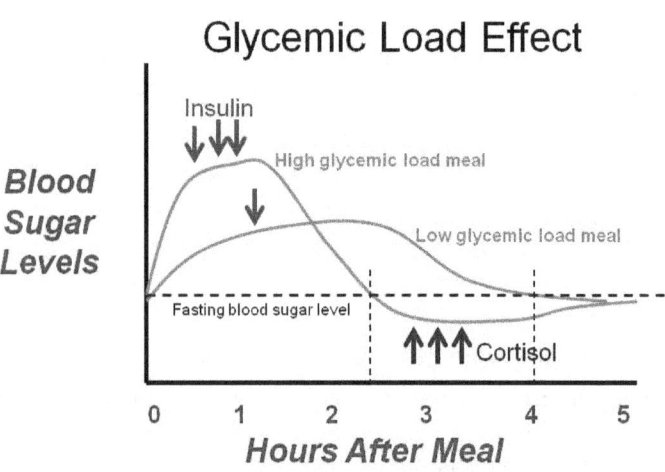

High Glycemic Food Metabolism

When you eat a high glycemic meal, there's an immediate rise in blood sugar. This sudden rise causes the body to put out high levels of insulin. This drops the blood sugar faster and can cause hypoglycemia.

Since the body's cells do not immediately require the sugar, the body forwards much of the sugar straight to the liver where it is converted for the storage of fat (triglycerides.)

The rapid drop of blood sugar level then leads to hunger and triggers the delivery of cortisol from the renal glands. This leads to deposits of fat in the abdomen.

Low Glycemic Food Metabolism

A low glycemic meal may contain the same number of calories and grams of sugars as a high glycemic meal - but because the low glycemic meal contains more fiber grams per sugar grams - it is slowly digested and absorbed.

The metabolic result is a very gradual rise in blood sugar, a much lower insulin output and the complete use of the sugars for energy: and because there is no excess sugar left over - there is no production of fat (triglycerides) from that low glycemic meal.

The glycemic index ranks food on a scale of 1 to 100 based on a measure of how fast blood sugar rises after a food is consumed. Foods with a glycemic index below 55 are considered low glycemic.

The gradual absorption of sugars over this same 4 hour period, illustrated above, sustains the energy levels needed for daily activities and suppresses the hunger response for a much longer interval.

Also, the adrenal glands are not stimulated to produce cortisol - when insulin and glucose (sugar) levels are low. Remember, these two meals contain the exact same grams of sugar and number of calories, yet they have much different effects on fat production and the hunger response. And it is all due to the low sugar/fiber ratio of the food.

Examples are whole grains, brown rice and legumes. Bad, or simple, carbs trigger a fast rise in

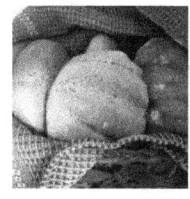

blood sugar. Some examples of bad or simple carbs are: white bread, refined pasta, processed cereals, cookies, candy and sugary sodas. Something to remember: a food that is significantly processed will spike your glycemic levels and lack a good source of fiber. Flour is used for many things but many don't realize the important vitamins and minerals are depleted, if not completely lost, as well as the fiber, when flour is refined.

The most common carbs that people consume aren't the good kind. In a typical diet among Americans, carbs make up 55% of their daily calorie intake.

To be a little more specific, sweet beverages, fruit juice and sugary sodas make up 10% of these calories. Refined bagels, cookies, muffins, cakes and white bread make up 20 to 25% of calories. Refined cereals, tortillas, potatoes and white rice make up 10 to 15% of calories. Only 5 to 10% of the calories are from healthful sources such as whole grains or non-starchy vegetables.

SUGAR (GLUCOSE), INSULIN AND INSULIN RESISTANCE (THE METABOLIC SYNDROME)

Insulin Resistance represents a major underlying abnormality driving most of our modern-day metabolic, inflammatory, medical diseases. These metabolic inflammatory medical diseases that have Insulin Resistance as the trigger also go by the name "the Metabolic Syndrome" as they all have inflamed (damaged) receptors and Insulin Resistance in common. Insulin Resistance (the metabolic syndrome) actually causes hyperinsulinemia and hyperglycemia ! And it is this excess circulating insulin and glucose that causes inflammatory damage to surrounding tissues and cells.

Some of these medical diseases triggered or caused by Insulin Resistance (hyperinsulinemia or hyperglycemia or both) are: type 2 diabetes, some cardiovascular, neurological, eye and kidney diseases as well as some cancers. These are the same medical diseases that are considered the major cause of morbidity and mortality in much of the world today.

A brief review of the history of the link between cardiovascular disease and insulin resistance includes a cluster of factors, including obesity, hypertriglyceridemia, hypercholesterolemia (atherosclerosis), hypertension and they all are associated with increased risk for coronary artery disease (CAD). It is this cluster of factors that are used to make the diagnosis of "the metabolic syndrome".

Note- Many diabetics are not only hyperglycemic but ironically they are also actually hyperinsulinemic: however, even though they are hyperglycemic and hyperinsulinemic the glucose cannot get through the damaged insulin receptor.

The components of the metabolic syndrome have increased scientific interest and excitement as well as the opportunities to investigate the links between insulin resistance and the many inflammatory metabolic diseases (e.g., cardiovascular disease, etc.), have multiplied.

If counting carbs, pay attention to net carbs. Counting carbs, not calories? Yes, you can count carbs in an easier fashion than counting calories, granted you know exactly where to look.

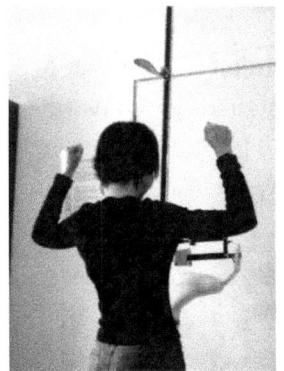

The first step is learning to identify which foods are already high in carbohydrates naturally. Such foods include starchy vegetables (potatoes, peas and corn), pasta, sweets, cereals, rice, and anything with sugar and flour.

Methods for counting your carbs might include the use of online carb counters and/or tables found in diet books targeted at low-carb eating. Look at the labels on packaged foods and calculate the total amount of 'net' carbs. To do this, locate the total grams of carbs per serving, and subtract the grams of sugar and fiber totals. For example, suppose a can of beans has 18 grams carbohydrates and 6 grams of fiber: the net carb amount would total 12 grams.

The body doesn't absorb the carbohydrates in fiber as it's non-digestible and sugar alcohol doesn't have many calories, (cookies, candy, etc.) so the body takes longer to absorb it and it slightly affects the blood sugar levels.

SUMMARY

In order to get off to a good start each and every morning, you should fill your stomach with food choices that are high in fiber, protein and micro-nutrients and low in sugars. Some good examples include oatmeal with blueberries, plain unsweet yogurt with fruit and walnuts, or eggs whites with 100% whole grain toast or cheerios with 2% milk or milk substitute.

The trick to recognizing a good whole grain: Use the carb/fiber ratio. Carbohydrates that contains adequate fiber generally do not affect your blood glucose levels which is why Low Carbohydrate diets often mention this concept of "net" carbs. Keep in mind that fiber containing carbohydrates have other effects on digestion. Finally, read labels, understand the sugar/fiber ratio and just use common sense.

WELL-KNOWN DIETS

Some of the well known diets include the Atkins diet, the Keto-Genic diet by Denise, the CG diet, the South Beach diet, the Mediterranean diet, The DASH diet. Other diets that fared well include: Weight Watchers, the Jenny Craig diet, the Medifast diet, the Chromium Picolinate diet, the Zone diet (40-30-30) which is more of a low fat - high carbohydrate diet (The Zone diet is not recommended any more by many physicians and nutritionists), Green Tea-Fat Burning diet, the Green Coffee Bean diet, the Dexatrim Max Complex diet, the Therapeutic Lifestyle Changes Diet, Garcinia Cambodia diet of Okinawans and the Alkaline diet of Hollywood, etc., to mention a few..

The most famous is the Atkins diet, which is almost identical to Denise's Keto-Genic Diet. They both start with an induction phase, a very-low-carb diet of fewer than 20 grams of carbohydrates daily, and then allow a few more carbs over the next 3 to 6 months. The South Beach diet more closely resembles the Atkins regimen but does not restrict carbohydrates as much in the early phase. Other low-carb diets are less strict. The Zone diet, also known as the 40-30-30 diet, is a calorically restricted diet that recommends that 40% of calories come from carbs, 30% from protein and 30% from healthful fats (ones that include omega 3 and omega 6 from plants and fish).

Note- "fasting" without prayer is and can be called dieting.

KETO-GENIC DIET by DENISE

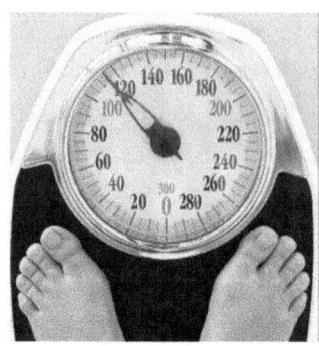

Menu: <u>Breakfast</u>: 2eggs any style, bacon, cheese (add a vinegar tablet or ½ grapefruit or ½ cup grapefruit juice). 1 to 2 cups Tea or Coffee [black - no sugar (no artificial sweeteners)].

<u>Lunch or Dinner/Supper</u>: Meat: beef hamburgers or steak, chicken, fish, pork, (broiled, baked or grilled): Salad with vinegar & oil – may have fruit and nuts on salad: Vegetables-raw or cooked in real butter or canola oil: 3 cups or glasses of un-sweet Tea or Black Coffee.

1. At meal time eat until you are full: this distends the stomach and stops the production of Ghrelin: a hormone that triggers the brain you are starving. Ghrelin is the hunger hormone.

2. Do not eliminate the "real fat" portions from this diet. Real fat does not form fat directly because it does not raise insulin. (Insulin is the fat storing hormone: Glucagon is the fat burning hormone.)

3. This diet completely eliminates simple carbohydrates and sugars: the real fat formers because they signal the pancreas to release a surge of - insulin: the fat storing hormone.

4. Grapefruit or vinegar tablets or dill pickles are an important aspect of this diet: These foods act as catalysts that start the fat burning process - (Lipolysis).

5. Do not eat deserts, breads, potatoes and white vegetables. These are considered high glycemic foods. They cause a surge in Insulin: which actually causes weight gain. You may double the helpings of meat or salad or other low-glycemic foods. Eat until you are full: but stay away from high glycemic foods.

6. You may snack on raw unsalted nuts or raw vegetables, etc. However, if you eat the combination of foods suggested you will not get hungry.

7. Drink 8 cups (8 oz) of unflavored water every day.   (This is ½ gallon of pure water).

Water neutralizes the sugar or sweet flavor on your tongue and thus decreases the production of a surge of insulin. Water also helps eliminate body waste faster preventing constipation. Constipation can interfere with healthy weight loss.

You may have: Broccoli, Carrots, Cabbage, Cole slaw, Cucumbers, Radishes, Spinach, Tomatoes, Lettuce, Nuts (no salt), Squash, Fried green vegetables, Green beans, Beans, Green apples, Grapes, Berries (black, blue or strawberries), Pears, Plums, Mangos, Mustard, Peppers, Real Dressing, Garlic and herbal seasoning, Tuna, Sardines, Salmon, Bacon, Meats, Chili (no beans), Cheese, Skim milk, and Hot Oatmeal with butter but no sweetener.

NOTE- Use Grapefruit or Grapefruit juice or Vinegar tablets or Dill pickles with each meal.

You may not have: Highly processed Cereal, Corn, Sweet Pickles, Jam or Jelly, Canned fruits in heavy syrup, Fruit Juices that contain artificial sweeteners and/or high fructose corn syrup, Diet Dressing,

Denise Marks, M.D.

White Onions, Peas, Pasta, Pretzels, Potatoes, Potato Chips, Corn Chips, Sweet Pickles, and all sweet desserts while on the Keto-Genic Diet.

This diet works best if you are will go on a "sugar-salt fast" the first two weeks. You can go off this recommended low glycemic diet – above- one day every other week and still lose weight.

The HCG Diet

The HCG diet was discovered quite by accident by Doctor A.T.W. Simeons over 50 years ago as he worked to cure malnutrition in underdeveloped villages. He discovered HCG, or human chorionic gonadotropin, the hormone, in pregnant women. He would observe the women's health throughout their pregnancy but noticed soon after childbirth that the health of the mother started to deteriorate. Obviously there had to be a reason for this occurrence.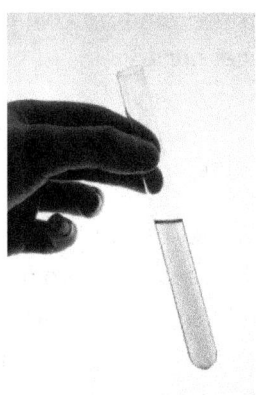

This is the moment HCG was discovered. HCG is a naturally occurring hormone that the body uses to protect and nourish the fetus by utilizing the fat reserves stored in the body, changing to provide the placenta with nutrition. People who are obese could actually benefit if this newfound discovery actually has the ability to drain fat cells and undergo a transformation that provides good, natural energy.

Three different types of fat are in the body: structural, normal reserve and abnormal. The fat located between your organs and skin is the structural fat and is important, as it is a protective layer of fat. When you aren't getting enough calories, your body will look for energy from the normal reserve fat. The fat you likely despise is the abnormal fat (a.k.a. 'extra' fat) typically found in the butt, thigh, hip, and waist regions. This is the fat that HCG consumes.

A question asked by many people, "So, if this is true, then why can't I achieve the same results on a low calorie diet?" First off, if your body isn't receiving the proper amount of vitamins and protein (as a low calorie diet may do), it will simply make up for that lack by using fat of any kind, including your normal reserve and structural fats. This in turn would start destroying your lean muscles and the fat you regain (because with a low calorie diet you *will* regain it), will automatically be abnormal fat. Bottom line? You didn't gain anything with a low calorie diet aside from simply distribute the existing fat.

There are three phases include in the HCG fat release program

(1) During the first phase you will build your fat reserves by eating whatever and how much you like for two complete days while starting the administering of the HCG drops.

(2) Phase two follows: For the next 23 to 40 days, a 500-calorie diet consisting of vegetables, fruits and two meals of 3.5 oz. of protein are followed while taking the HCG.

(3) Phase three is the maintenance part of the diet and a new way of living. Each as much as you want as long as starches and sugar are eliminated. Note- This is also the basis of the Atkins and Keto-Genic diets.

The reason for Phase 1 is to get the HCG circulating in the body before the regiment begins. After two days, the brain will have had ample time to know that the release of fat is to start. Adding to the fat reserves during this period is crucial by signaling the HCG of what process needs addressed.

As you enter into Phase 2 of the program, an average weight loss of 1 pound per day will be seen. You can continue for the amount of days that it takes to get to a desired weight. Going into Phase 3, continue

Denise Marks, M.D.

on the 500-calorie diet for two days to allow the HCG to completely leave your system. No more treatments should then be needed.

The time tested HCG protocol lets you enjoy naturally induced energy while reaping the benefits of weight loss. Your unneeded fat stores will be released into the blood stream and eliminated without a tinge of hunger.

Benefits of the HCG Diet

There are many benefits found in the HCG diet that are not found in fad diets.

- ❖ Slight increase and elevation in testosterone levels and metabolism
- ❖ Reduction in flabby or excessively fatty areas due to the redistribution of fat
- ❖ No worry of starving yourself from the lack of needed calories
- ❖ Burn fat without burning muscle
- ❖ Libido increase for both male and females
- ❖ Reduction in sweet-tooth cravings
- ❖ Affordable and easy program/plan to follow

HCG has actually been used for many years successfully by physicians and clinics. Some patients have even noticed life-changing results due to the combinations of hormone injections and a strict diet: people who were unsuccessful in other diet attempts. Unfortunately, at the time it was rather expensive to diet this way.

Nowadays, laboratories have created a natural homeopathically prepared medicine that doesn't require the use of medical supervision. Before, patients had to worry about the side effects. Now, thanks to small quantity manufacturing, people can avoid any unwanted side effects while taking HCG.

FDA has approved certain homeopathic HCG products for regulating PMS and as an aid for conception, but not exactly for *weight loss*.

More studies are being conducted on HCG and as time goes on, this could very well be added to the list of assets for HCG.

It's important that you don't start any kind of diet without first consulting with your physician. If you have an underlying medical problem you could experience adverse side effects from certain diets. Medical specialists have determined that HCG can be taken without worry of any serious side effects when taken with other medications. This includes birth control.

THE SOUTH BEACH DIET

Phase One: you should be eating six times per day, so it's important to think in terms of spreading your eating out over more smaller meals instead of fewer large ones. (This has the advantage of evening out your blood sugar as well.)

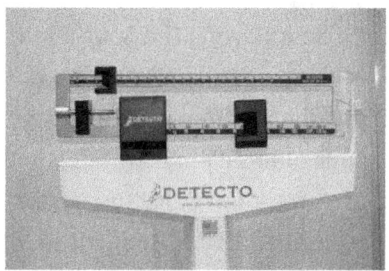

Breakfast
For breakfast you should have one serving of protein (like meat, tofu, cottage cheese or eggs) and one serving of vegetables (which includes vegetable cocktails like V8 and tomato juice). Your drink should be tea, coffee or anything calorie-free.

Dairy is the only food you have limits: the rest have no limits so if you aren't quite full, simply eat a little more of the aforementioned options.

Lunch
Your lunch should consist of one serving of protein (approved protein options with no serving size specified) and several servings of vegetables like beans. You could enjoy a chicken or tuna walnut salad

Denise Marks, M.D.

with just 1-2 tablespoons of dressing. Use cheese for your dairy and a calorie-free beverage like tea or water.

Dinner

Your dinner should have a serving of protein, several servings of vegetables and however much dairy you have left to eat, if you wish to have it at this time. Otherwise, it could be saved for dessert. 1-2 tablespoons of olive oil or other approved fat can be used in cooking or as a dressing. Top it off with a calorie-free beverage like water or tea with lemon.

Snacks

While following the South Beach Diet, you're allowed two snacks each day. An ideal snack on this diet would be something that provides both protein and vegetables. You might combine celery with your tuna salad or bean dip with raw veggies. Seeds and nuts are a preferred and delicious snack providing both fiber and protein but only a handful or ¼ cup of seeds would be ideal.

Desserts

Desserts aren't a requirement on the South Beach Diet, like snacks are. Most desserts approved during Phase One typically consist of ricotta cheese. In addition, you can have 75 calories of Truvia or Stevia each day.

THE MEDITERRANEAN DIET

I wouldn't necessarily call this a 'diet' rather than a mixture of the traditional eating habits of those residing in Greece, France, Italy, Spain and the Middle East.

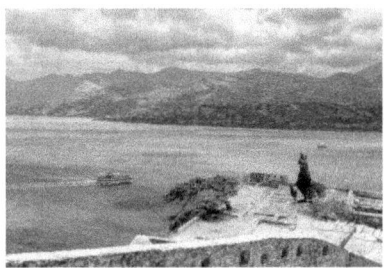

Benefits

There are actually quite a few scientists that believe the gold standard for healthy eating is following the Mediterranean Diet. Of course, the many studies being done regularly and appearing in the leading scientific journals prove the Mediterranean Diet can be a very healthy option for many.

Here are just some of the many examples of how these studies have confirmed the health benefits of the Mediterranean Diet.

- This diet alone can help reverse heart disease and lessen the risk for strokes.

- You can lower your cholesterol levels with the diet without the addition of medication.

- A diet low in sodium will help those who suffer hypertension.

- Losing weight safely and enjoying the long-term benefits of weight loss can be had while following the Mediterranean Diet.

- Avoid the need for diabetes drugs and help prevent diabetes while on the Mediterranean Diet.

- Many studies have shown that certain foods can alter estrogen levels. Dairy foods could also increase the risk for prostate cancer.

Denise Marks, M.D.

- Those who live in Mediterranean countries have fewer numbers of people with hip fractures.

- Improve cognitive capacity and lessen the risk for Alzheimer's with fruits and vegetables packed with antioxidants.

- The Mediterranean Diet can also help those suffering with IBS, frequent constipation, acid reflux, autoimmune diseases, blindness, and arthritis.

Starting the Mediterranean Diet.

- Eat natural, unprocessed foods like fruits, vegetables, whole grains and nuts.
- Make olive oil your primary source of dietary fat
- Reduce the consumption of red meat (Monthly)
- Eat low to moderate amounts of fish (Weekly)
- Drink a moderate amount of wine (up to one to two glasses per day for men and up to one glass per day for women)

Foods to Eat on the Mediterranean Diet

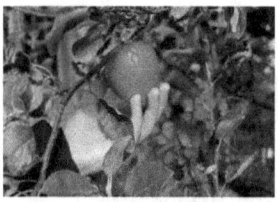

Fresh Fruit – It's important to eat a proper amount of fruit while on the Mediterranean Diet: 3 or 4 pieces are recommended. Consider oranges because they are a great source of antioxidants and phytochemicals: both helpful for disease prevention and protection. Antioxidant rich fruits are the best option so consider berries as well: blueberries, strawberries, etc. Protecting against cancer and heart disease is important and can be achieved with an antioxidant-rich diet. Most people who follow the Mediterranean diet consume their fruits for dessert.

Veggies – Salads are a common meal for Mediterranean's and lemon or olive oil is

68

typically used for the dressing. It also helps that both are packed with antioxidants. Another staple in this particular diet is tomatoes: including tomato products because they're a good source of antioxidants due to the lycopene they contain. Zucchini is another option to compliment your salad or sauté zucchini and cover with olive oil for a dressing.

Whole Grains – Whole grains are important and can be consumed in 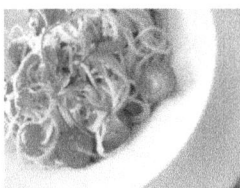 the form of bread, however you shouldn't combine a piece of whole wheat or grain bread with pasta meals. Choose whole wheat pasta and plan to eat this 2-3 times a week. It's a low-calorie option packed with fiber.

Beans – Legumes are important on the Mediterranean diet and include garbanzo beans, lentils and dried beans. You should eat them 2-3 times every week. According to the nutrition experts at Michigan State University you can actually lower your risk 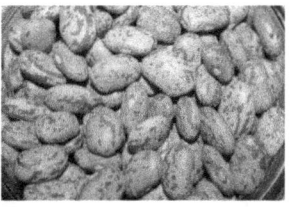 for heart disease by eating 2-4 cups of cooked legumes each week. The excess cholesterol in our bodies is eliminated by the fiber in dry beans. Animal protein puts a heavier load on our kidneys so opt for vegetable protein.

Nuts – Most everyone loves nuts, and just about any kind, but they 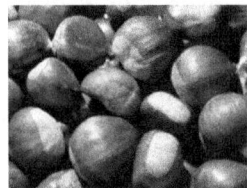 can actually be beneficial to incorporate into your diet. When you need a snack, consider a handful of nuts. Mediterranean countries actually consider nuts to be staple foods because they are a good source of monounsaturated fat: the kind that will not clog your arteries. Unfortunately, you will still need to eat them according to portion size due to their high calorie amounts. Walnuts and almonds are just two of the best options.

Denise Marks, M.D.

Olive Oil- The primary fat source in Mediterranean countries is olive

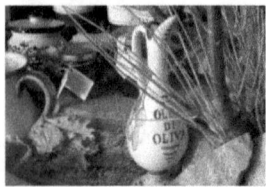

oil. It's used for both cooking and for dressing salads. It's the high intake of olive oil that can be contributed to the very low heart disease rate in those particular countries.

Seafood & Fish- When following the Mediterranean diet you will need to have seafood and/or fish 2-3 times every week. Sardines and salmon are packed with Omega-3 oils, which the body requires but does not produce enough on its own.

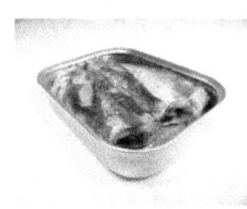

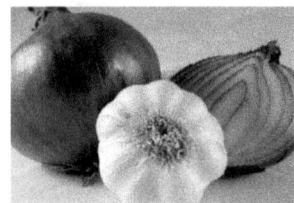

Aromatic Herbs & Garlic – The only condiments you will need are garlic and aromatic herbs. Garlic lowers blood pressure and can be confirmed by the blood pressure levels of those living in Mediterranean countries.

Sample Mediterranean Diet Menu

Like studies have shown, the 28 day diet plan for a Mediterranean diet will gradually introduce new changes that will lead to long-term changes. To begin, avoid any processed foods and increase your intake of vegetables and fruits. Next, add more beans to your weekly menu and opt for extra virgin olive oil (or others) instead of butter or other non-healthy oils. You will eventually reduce your red meat consumption to one portion a month, and you should only consume eggs, poultry and seafood a few times each week. Lastly, avoid milk, butter and cream and focus on ideal dairy choices.

Daily Meal Example:

Breakfast – A Greek yogurt with walnuts and fresh berries, tea or coffee to drink.
Lunch – Lentil soup with swish chard and taziki sauce

Snack – Cheese with whole grain crackers

Dinner – A serving of roasted cod with wheat berry salad and olive oil dressing, parsley, tomatoes and feta, with a glass of red wine, coffee, tea or water.

Dessert – Fresh fruit with a drizzle of honey

Losing Weight on the Mediterranean Diet

If you're like most, you are very curious how you will lose weight while on the Mediterranean diet: you aren't alone. Your diet will play an important role in the weight loss success.

Every day you should consume at least 5 servings of vegetables and fruits. Opting for those high in fiber, phytonutrients and vitamins is ideal. Plan to have beans (legumes) 8 times every week because they are packed with protein and fiber with low fat amounts. Opt for whole grains and avoid, if not limit, your refined grain intake. Choose low-fat dairy foods and have a tbsp of olive oil a day.

Have a maximum of two servings each of eggs, poultry and fish each week. They are packed with protein but possess higher calories. If you enjoy wine, have no more than one glass a day. Just 4 ounces of red wine packs a punch with antioxidants but also has up to 120 calories.

For dessert choose fruit, eat a maximum of two eggs each week, olive oil should replace your butter and honey to replace sugar. Red meat is only allowed one time a month and every day you will need to take part in thirty minutes of moderate physical activity.

Denise Marks, M.D.

AZTEC DIET

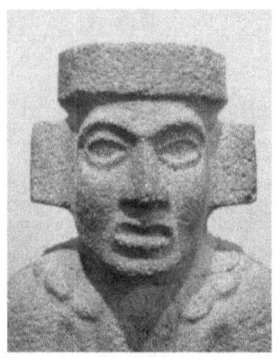

Normally Aztecs had two meals per day, and laborers got three meals, one at dawn, one at around 9 in the morning and another one at about 3 in the afternoon.

As with the food that Mexicans often eat today, Aztecs liked the spicy and rich food. They enjoyed <u>flavored maize, beans and squash with chili peppers and spicy sauces</u>.

The main food of Aztecs was the taxcalli -- a <u>corn-meal pancake</u> which was similar with the tortilla. Aztec food was commonly wrapped around meat and vegetables in order to make tacos. Their diet was mostly vegetarian, with turkey eggs and turkey meat.

Note- <u>Salvia hispanica, commonly known as chia</u>, is a species of flowering plant in the <u>mint family</u>, Lamiaceae, native to central and southern Mexico and Guatemala. . It is still used in Mexico and Guatemala, with the seeds sometimes ground, while whole seeds are used for nutritious drinks and as a food source.

Salvia hispanica is one of the two plants known as chia, the other being Salvia columbariae which is more commonly known as the golden chia. Chia is an annual herb growing to (3.3 ft) tall, with opposite leaves (1.6–3.1 in) long and (1.2–2.0 in) broad. Its flowers are purple or white and are produced in numerous clusters in a spike at the end of each stem. Chia is hardy from Zones 9-12.

Many plants cultivated as S. hispanica are actually S. lavandulifolia. Chia is grown commercially for <u>its seed, a food that is rich in omega-3 fatty acids</u>, since the seeds yield 25–30% extractable oil, including

72

(alpha) *a* linolenic acid (ALA). A chia seed is typically very little and oval shape and a 0.039 inch diameter. They are black, white, gray and brown.

Mexico is known for consuming the chia seed and some southwestern states in the U.S. as well. However, Europe is not too familiar with the chia seed. Salvia hispanica is how chia is often identified and is grown commercially today in Mexico, Bolivia, Ecuador, Guatemala, Australia, and Ecuador.

The largest producer of Chia was in Australia in 2008. Golden chia or salvia columbariae are similar species and used the same way but they are not commercially grown for food. Just one serving of chia seeds (1 oz: 28 g) has 5mg of sodium, 4g of protein, 11g of dietary fiber and 9g of fat, according to the USDA.

In regards to the recommended daily intake amounts, chia seeds amount for 18% calcium, 30% manganese, and 27% phosphorus of the daily intake recommendations. This same nutrient content is close to those of sesame and flax seeds.

There has been some preliminary research done to indicate chia could potentially offer benefits to dietary health, but unfortunately there is not enough evidence yet to fully support this claim.

Chia seed consumption has been reported in the public media and is purportedly used by athletes. Chia seeds may be added to other foods as a topping or put into smoothies, oatmeal, yogurt, made into a gelatin substance, or consumed raw. Also, chia seeds do not alter the taste of other foods if added to them.

Denise Marks, M.D.

DANIEL'S DIET

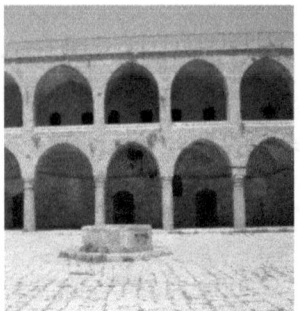 Daniel's diet starts with a Daniel's "fast". It is based on the "fasts" that are mentioned in the Holy Bible. There are two scriptures that advise two types of Daniel "fasts".

The first fast is based on 2 Kings 24 and the other is based on Daniel, chapter 1 and is considered Daniel's personal "fast". The 2 Kings 24 "fast" lasts for 10 days and you can eat only vegetables, fruits, nuts and seeds and drink only water.

Whereas, in Daniel's personal "fast" one needs to abstain from the "King's meal" for 21 days. The "King's meal" consists of meat, sweet breads and wine. For one to go on a "King's meal" fast they will need to abstain from all meat, all sweet breads and wine for 21 days. Other than the above mentioned foods, <u>one cannot eat any artificial or processed foods, foods with chemicals, yeast and baking powder.</u>

The Story Behind the Fast. In the Bible it is mentioned in Daniel, Chapter 1, that Daniel and some other children of Israel were held captive in Babylon. The good-looking, smart and quick learners of these captives were taken to the king's palace. Here, they were taught the Chaldean language and literature. Daniel and his companions were provided with the "King's meal" and wine daily.

Daniel rejected the foods that the King of Babylon set before him, and the principal court official got worried that this young man and others like him would become weak. The King would not be happy with this because these young men, along with several other Israelite captives, had been hand selected as the best of them all. He wanted them trained to serve in the palace.

At this time, Daniel made a request (as a test) to the court official,, to provide him and his companions a diet that included seeds, vegetables, fruits, nuts and water, for ten days.

Upon the arrival of the end of those ten days, the men were in better health than those who consumed the foods of the rich King. They then went forth with very high-standard positions within the King's court. Thus, this diet came to be known as Daniel's "fast". Basically, Daniel's "fast" supports healthy eating.

Daniel's diet or "fast" has become known as a religious fast. As with any religious fast, the Daniel "fast" involves denying the flesh to deepen the relationship between man and God. This is not a practice required by God, nor is it required by the church. It was and still remains a free-will offering to God intended to gain clarity in certain matters or strengthen the character of the individual undergoing the "fast".

What Food to Eat on a Daniel Diet (Fast)

You could look at this is a 'partial' fast, based on vegan cuisine. It only took a little bit of research to learn that Daniel actually consumed more than just water and vegetables. Nonetheless, it was a healthy diet based on water and whole foods.

Vegetables for the Daniel Diet: Artichokes, Asparagus, Beets,
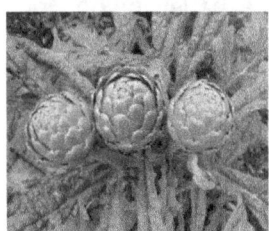
Broccoli, Brussels sprouts, Cabbage, Carrots, Cauliflower, Celery, Corn, Cucumbers, Eggplant, Garlic, Greens, Kale, Leeks, Lettuce, Mushrooms, Okra, Onions, Parsley, Potatoes, Peppers, Radish, Rutabaga, Scallions, Spinach, Sprouts, Squash, Sweet Potatoes, Tomatoes, Turnips, Zucchini.

Denise Marks, M.D.

Fruits for the Daniel Diet: Apples, Apricots, Bananas, Blackberries, Blueberries, Cherries, Boysenberries, Cantaloupe, Cranberries, Figs, Grapefruit, Grapes, Guava, Honeydew, Kiwi, Lemon, Lime, Mango, Nectarine, Oranges, Papaya, Peach, Pears, Pineapple, Plum, Raisin, Raspberries, Strawberries, Tangelos, Tangerines, Watermelon.

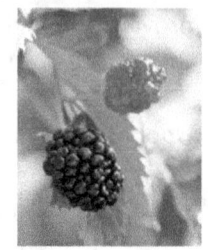

Other: In addition to the many vegetables and fruits, you should also have seeds and nuts, oats, barley and brown rice. Dried beans should be consumed often in addition to lentils and peas. If drinking water make sure it is spring or distilled and if you opt for vegetable or fruit juice, make sure it is 100% pure and free of additives. If you are worried about omitting any important nutrients, compliment your diet with a quality mineral and vitamin supplement.

Summary of Things You Can Eat on the Daniel's Diet.

It is actually somewhat confusing when it comes to determining what you can and cannot eat while on the Daniel fast. Here is a summary of different foods you can eat while on the diet:

- Fruits of all types: dried, juiced, canned, frozen and fresh.

- Vegetables of all types: juiced, canned, dried, frozen and fresh.

- Whole grains: whole wheat pasta, brown rice, barley, quinoa, rice cakes, oats, whole wheat tortillas, grits, millet and whole wheat.

- Nuts and Seeds: sesame, peanuts and peanut butter also.

- Legumes of all kinds including dried and canned.

- Natural oils: sesame, peanut, canola, grape seed, and olive.

- Pure or distilled water.

- Natural vegetable and fruit juices: no added sugar.

- Decaffeinated tea.

Other foods: herbs, spices, seasonings, soy products, salts and tofu.

Summary of Food to Avoid while on the Daniel's "Fast" Diet

While it's crucial that you know which foods are okay to eat, it's also important to know which foods to 'avoid' while on the Daniel fast. Such foods include:

- Deep-fried foods – lard, high trans-fats food, margarine, shortening.

- Sweeteners including white cane sugar and artificial sweeteners (including products that contain artificial sweeteners).

- All meat and meat products.

- Leavened bread and other bakery products.

- Refined and processed foods that contain artificial flavorings, preservatives, chemicals and food additives.

- Carbonated beverages, alcohol and energy drinks.

- Dairy products – butter, eggs, cream, cheese and milk.

The amount of food eaten should also be limited, preferably to only one meal a day. However, you may also take a vitamin supplement.

The Drink: Water should be the main beverage, (but only unsweetened water), 100-percent juice may also be consumed. It is

Denise Marks, M.D.

important to stay hydrated. Drink at least eight to ten glasses of water a day.

The Duration: The duration of the fast is up to the individual, and is dependent upon the intended result of the fast. The fast should be longer than a day, and can go for as long as the individual would like. Daniel originally participated in this fast for ten days and then continued for three weeks.

Warning: A medical evaluation should be done before undergoing the physical pressures of the any fast lasting longer than 3 days.

Note- You may experience a headache or joint pain near the beginning of the fast as the body is being purged of chemicals and toxins.

Daniel is an Old Testament prophet mostly known for being tossed out of the lion's den and emerging without a scrape. In his book, two fasts are mentioned that depict what was and was not eaten at that time. Many people, when seeking answers or determining which direction they should go regarding a certain situation, will refer to these fasts: also known as fasting. The first avoided foods that were offered to idols and the second was regarded with a time of prayer, mourning the condition of his people and Israel.

Tips for Fasting

- Because you are only allowed to eat certain foods it's important to ensure you get the right amount of nutrition.

- Roast vegetables, to get the most nutrition value, with lemon, honey, fresh spices of your choice (that has no additives, MSG, etc.), and pure extra virgin olive oil.

- Always keep leftover cooked rice easily accessible for times that you need a quick snack. Vegetables and fruit will digest quickly, likely causing you to be hungry again in a shorter timeframe.

- Visit your local farmer's or health market and purchase affordable carrots, tomatoes, celery and other goods to make healthy drinks if you have a juicer.

Eating fruits that naturally and safely lose weight will make you feel better overall while assisting to drop those extra pounds. Fruit helps you to lose weight because most are packed with fiber and essential vitamins and when eaten in place of less natural, wholesome foods they can really give you the advantage of shedding extra weight.

Foods to Avoid. Avoid the following foods if you attempt this fast:

- Meat
- White rice
- White flour
- Fried foods
- Caffeine
- Alcohol
- Carbonated drinks
- Refined sugar or sugar substitutes
- Fats, Margarine, Shortening
- Foods with preservatives or additives

When changing a diet that was once full of caffeine and other less wholesome products and food, it can wreak havoc on some people, as they will experience withdrawals. Luckily, it doesn't take long to rid these unhealthy things from your body and over time your body adjusts to your new diet.

Follow the Fast – When you are implementing a new diet plan it's important to stick to it all the way. This means you shouldn't veer from the approved foods and yo-yo or you won't achieve the weight

Denise Marks, M.D.

loss you're after. In addition, following the fast will help you achieve a balanced diet.

You shouldn't set your expectations too high and expect to lose a lot of weight while doing this fast. Fasting has a purpose and that is to move the heart of God by avoiding foods that most desire today in the world. This brings you closer to Him. Of course, it's important to pray as well when doing any fast.

THE ALKALINE DIET

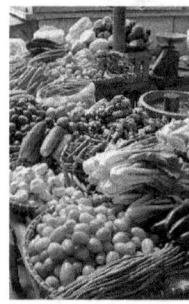

When our pH is too high or too low, we don't feel well, we feel tired, gain weight, have poor digestion and get aches and pains.

The alkaline diet has also been referred to as the alkaline acid or alkaline ash diet. The purpose of this diet is to encourage weight loss and prevent undesirable health problems like cancer, heart disease, arthritis, and diabetes. The reason being is that it's theory certain foods can actually produce acid which is not healthy and these foods include refined sugar, processed foods, wheat and meat.

The alkaline diet encourages you to eat foods that will make your own body more alkaline and protect against unwanted diseases and health concerns, while helping you to lose weight at the same time. You might remember hearing a lot about the alkaline diet when Victoria Beckham made a tweet regarding the cookbook for the alkaline diet back in 2013.

Is It Effective? Possibly, but likely for different reasons than it claims.

To begin with, to measure how acidic or alkaline something is, you go by the pH levels. Completely acidic foods will have a pH of 0, while something completely alkaline will have a pH of 14. Foods that are a pH level of 7 are considered neutral.

Your body will have various levels of pH throughout. A person's blood will be just slightly alkaline, measuring pH levels of anywhere from 7.35 to 7.45. It takes a lot for your body to keep it this way.

The stomach is considered to be very acidic with a pH level of 3.5 or less so that it can properly break down food. You have also likely noticed that your urine will change depending on your existing diet. This is how the body keeps pH levels in the body steady. The claim of the alkaline diet is that it can help the body maintain a balanced pH level at all times.

Because your body works very hard to keep this balance, there aren't any foods that will significantly alter the pH levels of your blood. It's also thought that you can achieve healthy weight-loss through the foods specific to this diet because they are alkalinizing.

Foods that you can eat while on the alkaline diet include significant amounts of vegetables, and lots of water as well as avoiding sugar, alcohol, colas, e.g., all soft drinks and processed foods and minimizing coffee, dairy, all meats and some fruits.

Other health claims, there's some early evidence that a diet low in acid-producing foods like animal protein (such as meat and cheese) and bread - and high in alkalinizing foods like fruits and veggies could **help prevent kidney stones, keep bones and muscles strong, improve heart health and brain function, reduce low back pain, and lower risk for colon cancer and type 2 diabetes**.

Those that fully believe in that the alkaline diet has to offer say you can achieve long-lasting acidity by shifting the blood pH levels

Denise Marks, M.D.

continuously, even though foods that produce acid only alter our pH balance for a short time.

You Can Have:

The majority of vegetables and fruits
Tofu
Soybeans
Legumes
Certain seeds and nuts

You Cannot Have:

Eggs
Most grains
Canned or Processed Foods
Packaged Snacks
Meat
Dairy
Convenient/Quick Foods

Not Recommended:

Soft Drinks (cola type)
Caffeine
Carbonated Beverages
Alcohol

THE VALUE OF CONSUMING ALKALINE FOODS

By ingesting more alkaline foods you are helping increase the amount of oxygen absorbed by the blood. Foods that are rich in alkaline include raw wheat grasses, unsweetened fruits, leafy green vegetables. Foods that are not considered alkaline are acidic foods. The amount of oxygen your blood absorbs can be measured through pH and ranges from 0-14.

Achieve an Alkaline Balance With the Right Acid

When we are slightly alkaline this means our blood is in balance with a pH level of 7.365. A great discovery was made at the start of the 20th century by intelligent scientists and winners of the Nobel Prize: we become ill when our blood isn't able to absorb the right amount of oxygen. Such illnesses include arthritis, diabetes, heart problems, Candida (yeast) infections, and even cancer.

You are likely aware that your body attempts to keep a steady, constant temperature of 98.5 degrees Fahrenheit. (37 degrees Celsius) However, are you aware that to maintain the proper balance of carbon dioxide/oxygen in your blood, the body has to put forth an even larger effort. If you aren't feeling well (weight gain, fatigue, digestion issues, pains, aches, etc.) it's likely because your pH levels are out of balance (too low or too high).

Did You Know? The majority of people in Europe and the United States are too acidic? Their bodies do not get enough oxygen in the blood. This is when you begin to see arthritis, diabetes, cancer and heart disease come in to play.

How Does a Person Become Too Acidic?

- Parasites
- Toxins
- Stress
- Food (that you eat)

LIST OF FOODS THAT ARE ACIDIC

Unfortunately, the majority of the foods that you absolutely love, are more acidic than you are aware, thus having a bigger impact on your health than you may realize. What might these foods be? They include:

- Processed Foods
- Junk Foods
- Sugar
- Unhealthy Fats (margarine, shortening)
- Animal Foods (chicken, lobster, meat, fish, eggs, oysters)
- Carbonated Beverages/Soft Drinks (Mtn. Dew, Dr. Pepper, Sprite, Cola, etc.)
- Grains – ((white) wheat, pasta, bread, flour, rice, etc.)
- Processed Drinks (especially juice drinks)
- Dairy – (butter, cheese and milk)
- Cashews, Peanuts
- Certain Fruits

THE ALKALINE FOOD LIST

We don't realize that most of the food we eat during the majority of our lifetime are rather high in acidic. They are what make us tired and feel sick. Our bodies can easily heal itself from many diseases simply by consuming alkaline drinks and raw alkaline foods.

What foods are considered alkaline? They include:

- Wheat Grass
- Fresh Spice and Herbs (cayenne, parsley, ginger, cilantro, basil)
- Sprouts (broccoli, mung bean, alfalfa, etc.)
- Fruits (cucumber, young coconuts, avocado, watermelon)
- Vegetables (preferably the raw leafy green variety)

What drinks are alkaline? The best options include:

- Young Coconut Water
- Wheatgrass Juice
- Alkaline Water
- Vegetable Juice

If your body is highly acidic it might be best to use an alkaline supplement to achieve a normal balance faster.

How Can I Tell if I'm Highly Acidic?

Are you curious what your own acidic levels are? Do you know your body's pH level? If not, don't worry, it's actually quite simple to determine your own alkalinity. You can purchase specific pH test strips at most health stores. You then pee on the strips and it will display your pH level, thereby telling you just how acidic your body is.

DETOXIFICATION DIET

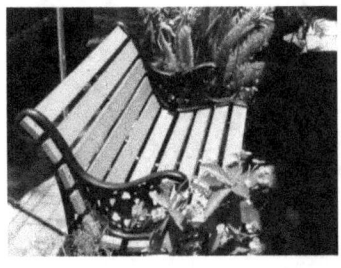

Detoxification has been practiced for centuries by many cultures around the world, including Jews and Christians alike as well as the Chinese medical systems. <u>Detoxification works because it addresses the needs of individual cells.</u> Studies show that everyone would benefit if they detoxed at least once a year. <u>Even a short detoxifying program that just cleanses the liver is beneficial for health</u>.

A full Detoxification diet is about resting, cleaning and nourishing the body from the inside out. Detoxification enhances the body's own natural healing systems. By removing and eliminating toxins from the blood, then feeding your body with healthy nutrients, detoxifying can

Denise Marks, M.D.

help protect you from disease, even many cancers and renew your ability to maintain optimum health.

 It does this mainly by removing impurities from the blood via the liver, where toxins are detoxified.

The body can then eliminate these "detoxified (neutralized) toxins" through the kidneys, intestines/colon, lungs, lymph and skin. However, when any of these systems are compromised, toxins aren't properly detoxified and every cell in the body is subjected to injury, inflammation and disease.

 Toxins are harmful (poisonous) substances and are obstacles to your health and natural healing processes. In order to prevent many of our modern day medical diseases it is necessary to maintain a healthy liver free of sludge.

A detox diet can help your liver's natural cleaning process and eliminating toxins by:

1) Resting your liver, first, through a form of fasting:

2) Stimulating your liver to detoxify:

3) Promoting the elimination of these toxins through the intestines, kidneys and skin:

4) Improving the circulation of the blood:

5) Refueling the body with healthy nutrients.

Remember, your body doesn't detoxify you - it is your liver that detoxifies your body. The liver uses enzymes, vitamins, minerals, anti-oxidants, and anti-inflammatory nutrients to neutralize free radicals. And it is these free radicals that cause most of our medical diseases.

There are many detoxification diets, recipes and programs that depend on your individual needs. There are several programs that stick to a 7-day schedule to ensure the body has enough time to cleanse the blood. When partaking in such a program you might expect to fast on liquids only for two days, with a 5-day 'detox' diet following to give the digestive system time to rest Also, herbs, supplements, low stress exercises, and practices such as dry-skin brushing and hydrotherapy are recommended.

A 3-7 day juice fast is a very strict and effective way to reduce toxins and is considered a very severe form of detoxifying. It involves drinking only fresh fruit and vegetable juices (especially celery and carrot juice) and water.

 Other popular detoxifying programs and natural body cleanses include: 1. Cleansing supplement packages, which generally contain fiber, vitamins, herbs and minerals. There are several safe products on the market. 2. A routine of drinking only water one day each week — an ancient practice of many cultures. Drinking only water for one day was a form of fasting in Biblical times.

YOUR LIVER IS RESPONSIBLE FOR DETOXIFING YOUR BODY.

Detoxification is one of the many functions of the liver. Remember: The liver combines toxic substances, such as drugs, alcohol, metabolic waste and environmental toxins with substances such as anti-oxidants, anti-inflammatory nutrients, vitamins and minerals that are not toxic to produce a neutralized substance. This neutralized substance is then excreted through the skin, kidneys and/or intestines (bowel). Certain nutritional drinks and/or foods help cleanse and maintain the liver and then heal many important functions needed by the body to heal and maintain good health.

The best way to get healthy is to work from the inside out starting with the cleansing (detoxification) of the liver. Putting the proper

Denise Marks, M.D.

nutrients into your body is always important, but first you want to flush out the toxins.

Toxic chemicals are really poisons. Remember, toxic chemicals cause many of our modern day medical diseases. The toxins that build up in the body are usually noticed first in your skin, causing it to look rough and dull: your body will begin to look puffy and then a disease process begins.

If your system is clean and free of toxic, poisonous chemicals that

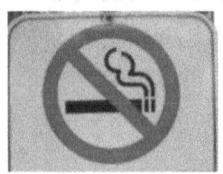 inflame and therefore cause cell damage: then and only then can the good nutrients you put into your body finally get to where they belong. When this finally happens then and only then can you be more energetic, beautiful and

healthy. There are many everyday natural foods that are great for detoxifying. **To begin a detox diet you will first need to reduce your toxin load**. To do this you will need to eliminate alcohol, coffee, cigarettes, refined sugars, especially high fructose corn syrups and artificial sweeteners as well as saturated fats, especially foods that contain trans-fats.

Trans-fats are found in nearly all processed foods on the market today. Trans-fat is another name for hydrogenated oils (margarine, shortening, etc.). And trans-fats are in any food made with these hydrogenated oils. This includes mayonnaise, some ice creams most cookies and/or nearly all processed baked goods. All of the above processed food products contain toxins.

Also, a detox diet works best if you minimize stress. Stress triggers your body to release stress hormones into your system. These hormones, in large amounts, can not only create toxins but also slow down the detoxification enzymes in the liver.

Along with detoxifying your body through diet, it is good to reduce stressful life situations. Yoga, some low stress exercises and meditation are simple and effective ways to relieve stress by resetting your physical and mental reactions to the inevitable stress life will bring.

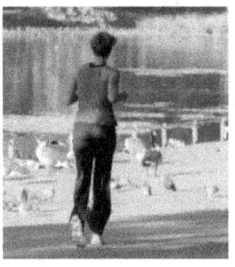

Foods that are known to help the liver detoxify free radicals:

*Celery and/or celery juice. The road to detoxification and therefore the road to healing may start with consuming celery juice. Celery juice is a good one to start with because celery juice has "natural" sodium, i.e. the same content of sodium as human blood (0.09%). If the saline level in your body is not hydrated you can become dehydrated causing hypernatremia: or over-hydrated causing hyponatremia. The salt in celery helps our bodies utilize the nutrients that are put into it.

The sodium in celery is organic and good for our bodies. Celery

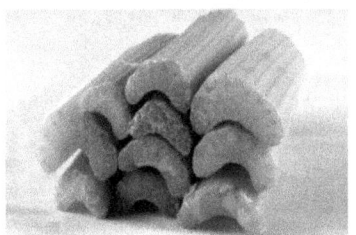

deletes carbon dioxide from the body and thereby regulates or counteracts the acid build up in the body. Celery has a great deal of fiber that helps control the absorption of dietary sugars and cholesterol thus controlling the blood sugar and cholesterol levels. Celery also helps the body to regulate temperature.

Celery is also good for the colon (digestive system) because it is also a colon cleanser. The nutrients in celery can also stimulate the elimination of urine from the body, and therefore celery acts as a diuretic. Celery is also a calming agent that is good for treating anxiety or other nervous disorders. Celery has been used for its medicinal powers for centuries. It is best to juice celery. However, celery is good cooked in soups and stews or eaten raw in salads. Celery is a food that basically brings the body back to normal.

* Warm Lemon Water: Lemons are a super-food rich in potassium, vitamin C and citric acid. Hot water and lemon, (a lemon tonic), has long been used as a staple in dietary programs for its positive effects on the liver, bile and digestion. Drinking warm lemon water can help cleanse the liver.

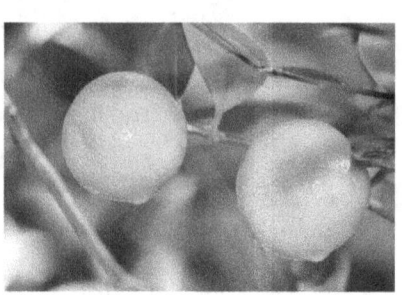

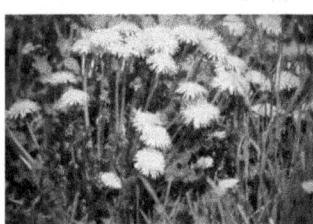

*Dandelion Tea: Dandelion contains nutrients, such as calcium, magnesium, iron, selenium, zinc, phosphorous and vitamins B and Dandelions can be boiled into a therapeutic tea that helps cleanses the liver.

*Fruit Smoothies: certain fresh fruits help to stimulate energy flow through the liver, enhancing its function. Blackberries, strawberries, blueberries, raspberries, gooseberries are considered good liver detoxing agents. NOTE- These healthy and potent berries make a delicious liver cleansing fruit smoothie when combined with other fruits, i.e., banana, and/or green leafy vegetables, i.e., spinach and almond milk.

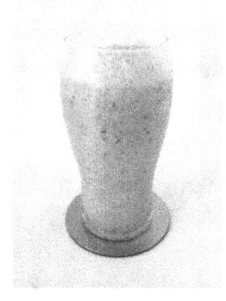

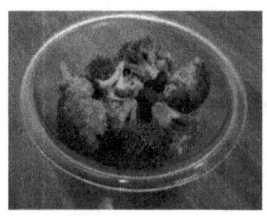

*Broccoli And Cabbage Juice: Broccoli and cabbage are cruciferous vegetables that can be juiced into a cleansing liver drink. Cruciferous vegetables are a rich indoles source. These vegetables include Brussels sprouts, broccoli, bok choy, cabbage and turnips.

Increasing your cruciferous vegetable intake is not recommended if you have a thyroid disorder. Cruciferous vegetables are known as goitrogens, which are foods that can suppress thyroid function. Note-eating a diet rich in fruits, vegetables and cereal grains may help to reduce your risk of cancer as well as other diseases.

*Bananas: Another example of a nutritious medicinal food is the

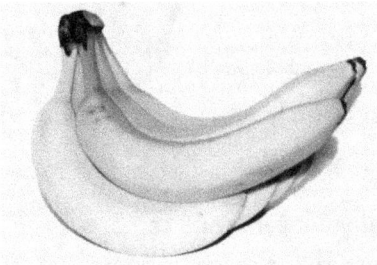

banana. Bananas are one of the most popular foods and for good reason. Bananas are filled with Potassium: giving your body the ability to handle stress, maintain a healthy blood pressure and provide sustained energy - the healthy way without any harmful side effects.

*Nutmeg can also clean your liver and kidney and remove many toxins. Just add nutmeg to as many fruit and milk drinks as you can. You can also add a dash of cinnamon.

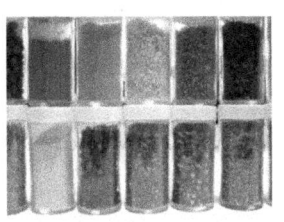

A Fruit & Veggie Flush is a 3 day diet that is considered both a detox diet and a weight loss diet that is considered safe for losing 8 to 10 pound. This diet should not be continued after 3 days. During these 3 days, you will only eat fruits and vegetables and drink lots of water: you'll lose weight and conquer food addiction. Basically, this vegetarian diet is really a jump-start diet to a safe and effective weight loss program that includes moderate

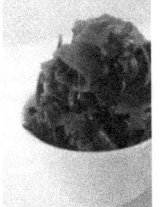

exercise.

*Seaweed . Seaweed contains a variety of nutrients and minerals, making it an excellent detox food choice.

91

Denise Marks, M.D.

Harmful toxins are removed from the body when they bind with the nutrients.

* Garlic. A well-known blood purifier, garlic is high in detox properties due to the antioxidants it contains. Garlic is also known as a natural cholesterol lowering supplement.

* Apple Cider Vinegar. Long used for its purifying properties, apple cider vinegar is a natural way to purify your body.

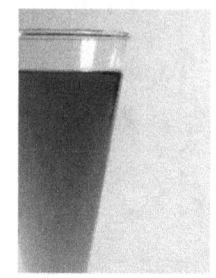

Not only does apple cider vinegar help your body detox, it also supports your immune system, helps control weight and promotes good digestion.

* Spirulina. The spirulina contains many nutrients and can boost nutrition during a detox phase. Dried spirulina contains about 60% (51–71%) protein. It is a complete protein containing all essential amino acids. It is superior to typical plant protein, such as that from legumes.

* High Fiber Raw Fruits and Veggies. Raw fruits and veggies are excellent purifying foods due to the amount of fiber they contain. Fiber is incredibly cleansing when it comes to the digestive system. Many people do not get near enough fiber

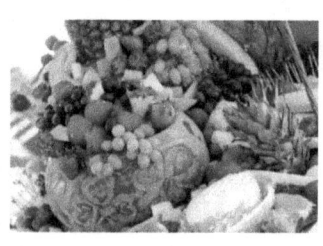

in their daily diet. High fiber fruits and veggies include: apples, arugula, bananas, blackberries, blueberries, carrots, figs, kale and strawberries.

The following are seven key principles to obtain optimal health.

1. Drink 6 to 15 cups (2 to 4 quarts) of pure water daily.

2. Minimize salt intake and maximize your potassium intake.

3. Eat the right types of fats, i.e., omega 3 fatty acids in fish or 1 to 3 grams of fish oil a day

4. Eat limited amounts of meat. Avoid processed meats.

5. Reduce your exposure to pesticides, both internal and external exposure.

6. Eat a wide variety of colorful fruits and vegetables.

7. Get at least 25 to 30 grams of fiber each day.

8. Eat low glycemic carbohydrates (complex carbohydrates) to regulate your blood sugar level.

9. Avoid drinks containing artificial, non-nutritive sweeteners or high fructose corn syrup.

Note- The main strength of a Fruit and Veggie detox diet is that it encourages you to eat fresh fruits and vegetables, which are an essential part of a healthful diet.

During a 3 day Fruit and Veggie detox program you will need to:

Drink at least 12 glasses of bottled or filtered water each day

Avoid non-water beverages, including coffee and tea

Eat any type of fresh veggie or fruit (no frozen, dried, or canned fruits), preferably organic

Have salad in the evening — all non-starchy, preferably organic, vegetables

Avoid strenuous exercise while on the 3 day program

Denise Marks, M.D.

THE DASH DIET

The dash diet has been named the best diet by U.S. News and World Report. A panel of experts evaluated 25 diets and chose the best weight loss program based on several factors. According the Los Angeles Times these included seven different 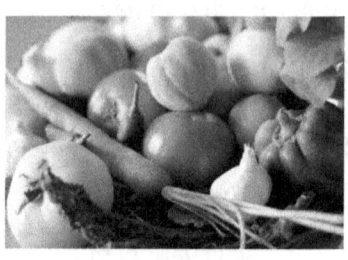 health-related criteria as well as "how well they generated short- and long-term weight loss."

Dietary Approaches to Stop Hypertension (DASH) is a government-endorsed program designed to fight high blood pressure. Dieters on the program eat foods that are low in sodium including plenty of fresh fruits and vegetables, whole grains, lean protein and low-fat dairy products. While the program was designed to fight hypertension, it is also very effective for weight loss.

If you find yourself diet shopping, the DASH Diet is a good place to start. But be sure to evaluate several weight loss plans before choosing the best diet for you. Often, what works for one dieter may not work for another. And if you are not quite ready to commit to a full-scale diet, there are still small changes you can make to improve your health.

CALORIES IN SUGAR

One cup of sugar is equal to 200 grams, which is 800 calories.

Can you even imagine eating 1 full cup of sugar every day?

Many people do without ever realizing it. If you drink 4 sodas (16 oz) in one day, you've drank almost a cup of sugar!

One (16 oz) cola drink contains 40 grams of sugar.

40 grams x 4 colas equal 160 grams of sugar daily.

One gram of sugar = almost 4 calories.

160 grams x 4 colas = 640 calories of sugar in one day.

Many processed fruit drinks contain as much or more sugar than carbonated beverages. Just because a drink is labeled "fruit drink" doesn't make it healthy!

Note also: one 16 oz high fructose corn syrup drink (cola as well as processed juices and sweet tea) contains 40 grams of sugar.

Remember: One teaspoon of sugar equals 4 grams (16 calories).

APPENDIX #1 HEALTHY THINGS YOU CAN DO TO MINIMIZE THE SUGAR SPIKE WHEN CONSUMING FOODS THAT HAVE A HIGH AMOUNT OF SUGAR per AMOUNT OF FIBER

1. Drink plenty of natural water, unsweet tea or coffee. Unsweetened drinks actually dilute the sugar content of cookies, cake or candy, thus reducing the rapid absorption of sugar and the resulting surge of insulin that would have occurred if it the sugar content was not diluted.

2. Dilute all fruit juices, including natural unprocessed fruit juice, with water. This reduces the rapid absorption of sugar and the resulting surge of insulin into the blood stream.

3. Add lemon or lime slices to water or tea. This is said to slightly alkalinize or neutralize the blood. Acidic blood is known to trigger inflammation.

4. It is better to eat protein with your carbohydrates than to eat fat-laden foods with carbohydrates (sweets). For example, oatmeal with sugar is better than toast with butter and jelly. That is because oatmeal contains more protein than toast.

5. Increase your activity. Exercise is known to bring one's blood sugar level down quickly thus reducing the surge of insulin. Exercise is a very important part of managing your blood sugar and insulin levels.

6. Successful healthy diet factors include: a healthy amount of protein, lots of fiber per carbohydrates (or sugar), fewer sugar calories, and limited saturated fat, with proportions tailored to your individual health profile, i.e., active vs. sedentary life styles.

7. If you have a sweet tooth, find healthy desserts. There are many healthy dessert recipes available online and in print.

APPENDIX #2 HEALTHY DESSERT IDEAS

Most desserts are full of sugar and fat. The extra carbohydrates and fats that are consumed when eating desserts can elevate your blood glucose and insulin, which hinder your weight-loss attempts and trigger or cause most metabolic medical diseases. However, by picking the right kind of desserts and limiting your portions, you can satisfy your sweet tooth and still keep your blood sugar and insulin requirements under control. The key is to keep track of your carbohydrates and fiber and incorporate healthy desserts as one part of your overall diet plan.

Remember, all foods that contain carbohydrates, such as all processed foods as well as natural unprocessed breads, cereals, fruits, vegetables, and milk, can affect blood sugar, not just desserts.

Note- The best way to incorporate a dessert into a healthy diet is to have it at the end of your meal. You can subtract main-meal carbs to make room for some dessert carbs. For example, have a 3-ounce portion of lean meat and fill half your plate with non-starchy vegetables like green beans or summer squash. Subtract the carbohydrates you would've gotten from rice, pasta, or potatoes and replace those carbs with a small dessert."

Some tips on choosing healthy desserts:

- ✓ Consume fresh fruit. Eating fruit for dessert can help you reach the recommended three to five servings per day.

- ✓ Choose dairy wisely. Use cheese, cottage cheese with fruit and/or 2% milk or plain Greek yogurt with chocolate.

- ✓ Exercise portion control. Always go for small portions or ask for extra spoons and share desserts with others.

Denise Marks, M.D.

- ✓ Consider sugar-free desserts made with Truvia. (If you choose sugar-free desserts note that the labeling can be misleading. Ignore the words on the front of the box and check the label on the back. Many so-labeled 'sugar-free' desserts actually contain a lot of carbohydrates and calories.

- ✓ Try individually wrapped ice cream treats with less than 30 grams of carbohydrates in place of ice cream that you have to serve yourself.

- ✓ Put half of a banana on a Popsicle stick, dip it in dark chocolate, and freeze it on wax paper.

- ✓ Meringue cookies can also be a good low-carb, low-fat option.

- ✓ Chocolate-drizzled peanut butter cake contains 193 calories and 23 grams of carbohydrates.

- ✓ Apple crisp parfait contains 149 calories and 35 grams of carb.

- ✓ Mango-ginger sorbet contains 110 calories and 29 grams of carb.

- ✓ A crispy oatmeal-raisin cookie contains 98 calories and 17 grams of carb.

While you don't need to give up sweets, counting grams of fiber and grams of sugar (carbohydrates), limiting saturated fats, and controlling portion sizes will help you enjoy desserts on any healthy diet.

Your basic goal will need to be: (1) watch your blood sugar levels and (2) maintain a healthy weight!

"Whole grain" has become a healthy eating buzz phrase, and food companies aren't shy about using it to entice us to buy products.

Last year, nearly 3,400 new whole-grain products were launched, compared with just 264 in 2001. And a poll by the International Food Information Council showed that 75% of those surveyed said they were trying to eat more whole grains, while 67% said the presence of whole grains was important when buying packaged foods.

Many of the products we buy may not deliver all the healthy whole-grain goodness we're expecting. If sugary Froot Loops can tout itself as a whole-grain food, there's something wrong with our advertising system.

WHAT'S THE BEST WAY TO IDENTIFY A HEALTHFUL WHOLE-GRAIN FOOD?

There are several competing recommendations. It's recommended by the Dietary Guidelines for Americans to select grain foods that are 'whole' above all other grains on the ingredient list. When looking at grain products, if the ingredient's list first item isn't whole grain, they do not recommend it. In addition, if it doesn't contain a 'whole' grain ingredient first and also has added sugars, they do not recommend it.

You've likely seen the Whole Grain Stamp on certain food products in the store and this is a promotion of the non-profit Whole Grains Council. They stamp a product if it has a minimum of 8 grams of whole grains, per each serving.

APPENDIX #3 NUTRIENTS IN ANTI-INFLAMMATORY FOODS

Foods Containing Anti-Inflammatory and Anti-oxidant Nutrients Are Also Considered to be Natural Medicines as well as Anti-Cancer Foods

Nutrients in Anti-inflammatory foods are the key to living a longer and a healthier life. These food nutrients are to help prevent as well as fight cancer. They are also considered **anti-aging food nutrients**. Basically, inflammation is a normal and essential part of our body's defense system. It is a natural way in which our body reacts to an infection, irritation or other injury. Also, inflammation refers to a set of biological processes involving the natural reaction of our body to harmful stimuli, i.e. injuries, infections, free radicals, toxins, etc.

Inflammation is the body's attempt at healing or repairing the damage caused by harmful foreign agents. It does this by removing the harmful stimuli, i.e., free radicals, irritants, toxic agents, pathogens (agents of infection), damaged cells and even abnormal precancerous cells.

Exposure to any of the above mentioned stimuli is basically inevitable in our daily lives. However, our body's natural defense can neutralize or fight most of the harmful (toxic) agents, to some extent, on its own when supplied with the right nutrients. Anti-inflammatory foods supply our body with the correct nutrients that help our body's natural healing processes that prevent and/or fight most of the modern-day, inflammatory, metabolic medical diseases.

Note- Inflammation does not mean infection, even when an infection causes inflammation. Infection is caused by a bacterium, virus or fungus, while inflammation is the body's response to it, the infectious agent or toxic or foreign chemicals.

Signs and symptoms of the damage caused by inflammation are swelling redness increased temperature, pain, tumors (benign and cancerous) and damaged receptors. Damaged receptor do not work properly (i.e., insulin resistance is the result of damaged receptors). If there aren't enough anti-inflammatory food nutrients consumed to correct the damage caused by this most often necessary biological response to foreign, harmful substances, then some or all of the symptoms above can increase to the point of causing many modern-day inflammatory diseases such as, diabetes, health disease, kidney and eye diseases, neurological and psychological diseases, many cancers, etc., that lead to death.

Inflammation basically can be acute (short term) or chronic (long term). Acute inflammation is a sign that the body is trying to heal itself and last within a 24 hour period of time. Chronic inflammation refers to what happens in our body over a longer period of time.

Chronic long term damage happens when our body's natural defenses (mainly our immune system, digestive system, cardiovascular system, etc.) are <u>overwhelmed</u> by the continuous exposure to harmful stimuli, which then renders our body and its natural defenses weak and unable to prevent, correct, fight, etc., further damage and disease.

Some examples of most of the common chronic metabolic medical disorders caused by inflammation are: Arthritis, Dermatitis, Gastrointestinal disorders, Neurological disorders, Cardiovascular disorders (Hypertension, Hypercholesterolemia, Hypertriglyceridemia, Atherosclerosis, Angina, Heart Attack, Stroke, etc.), Chronic Renal (Kidney) disorders, some Eye diseases, Diabetes, Obesity, Inflammatory Bowel Diseases, some Cancers, Aging Processes, and Auto-Immune diseases (those diseases that result when our body's defense mechanisms start attacking itself).

Denise Marks, M.D.

The following is a list of the most common anti inflammation and anti-oxidant foods by groups. Anti-inflammatory and antioxidant nutrients are also known as phytonutrients. These nutrients can slow down the aging process and prevent and/or treat and repair the internal injury or damaged tissues and cell receptors.

1. Vegetables: fresh or frozen, are basically anti inflammatory foods. The best examples include cruciferous vegetables that are exceptionally rich in a specific phytonutrient, the <u>sulphoraphanes</u>.

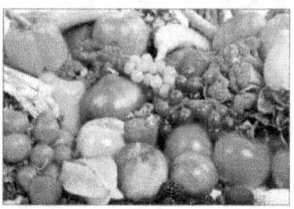

This phytonutrient is known to have <u>anti-cancer properties</u> as well as Spinach, a food that is rich in: vitamin B9 (folate), as well as minerals such as calcium, iron, magnesium, potassium, and phytonutrients such as carotenes, flavonoids and tryptophan.

Beets (contain boron)	Bell Pepper	Bok Choy
Broccoli	Cauliflower	Carrots
Chard	Egg plant	Fennel bulb
Green beans	Kale	Leeks
Mushrooms	Olives	

Onions, especially the spring onions

Salad greens	Shallots	Squash

Sweet potatoes (contains fiber, vitamin C and B6, beta carotenoids, manganese and carbohydrates).

2. Fruits: fresh or frozen, have both antioxidant and anti-inflammatory nutrients that are effective in preventing a number of diseases such as: arthritis, cancer, indigestion, acid peptic disease, dementia and many other chronic inflammatory conditions.

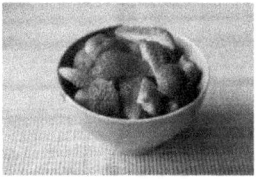

Apples (contain quercetin)

Avocados (contains omega-3 fatty acids which are natural anti-inflammatory agents)

Blackberries contain flavonoids (anti-inflammatory) and antioxidants (vitamin C)

Blueberries

Cherries

Gooseberries

Grapefruit (contains hesperidin and naringin, nutrients that block the internal production of cholesterol)

Grapes

Kiwi fruit

Lemons (Contains hesperidin)

Limes

Mangoes

Oranges (contains Hesperidin)

Papaya (contains papain, an enzyme known to aid in digestion of proteins)

Peaches (contain both anti-oxidants that neutralizing charge oxygen radicals and flavonoids that are known as super anti-inflammatory nutrients)

Denise Marks, M.D.

Plums

Pineapple (contains Bromelain)

Raspberries

Rhubarb

Strawberries

3. Fish and/or Fish Oils are considered to contain both anti-oxidant and anti-inflammatory agents. These fish are an excellent source of omega-3 fatty acids. These omega-3 fatty acids include eicosa-pentaenoic acid (EPA) and docosa-hexaenoic acid (DHA).

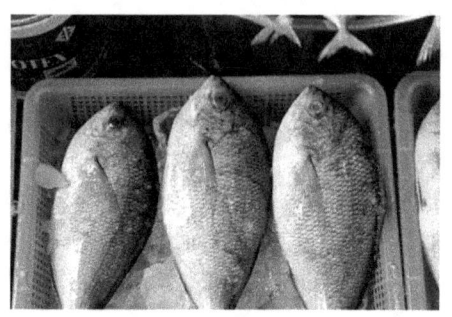

There are numerous benefits of omega-3 fatty acids some of which are: a healthier heart by reducing the chances of heart diseases, preventing and fighting cancer, helping prevent autoimmune diseases and psychological / neurological disorders. All of these benefits result from omega-3's excellent anti oxidant and anti-inflammation properties.

Cod	Halibut	Herring	Oysters
Salmon	Sardines	Snapper	Striped Bass
Tilapia	Trout	Tuna	Whitefish

4. Edible oils: of which the best three are Olive oil, Coconut oil and Avocado oil. These are considered to be excellent sources of anti-inflammatory nutrients, i.e. polyphenols and unsaturated fats.

Olive oil contains an abundant supply of polyphenols and monounsaturated fats, which reduce inflammation in cardiovascular system including heart and blood vessels, which in turn reduces the risk of atherosclerosis and all the resulting complications. It also helps prevent as well as treat Rheumatoid and Osteoarthritis and asthma caused by and allergic or autoimmune mechanism.

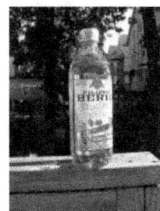

Avocado oil is the other edible oil that is considered a very effective anti-inflammatory agent. Avocado oil has similar properties to that of Olive oil.

Coconut Oil is another edible oil that is considered a very effective anti-inflammatory agent. Coconut Oil is a short chain saturated fat.

5. Drinks

Green tea is the best example of a drink that is rich in flavonoids, and contains very potent anti-inflammatory nutrients. Green tea also contains various anti-oxidants. These nutrients are known to decrease the incidence of cardiovascular (heart) diseases,

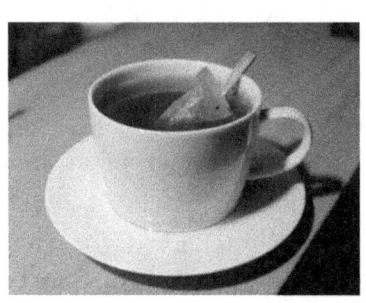

diabetes, arthritis, kidney and eye diseases, neurological disorders as well as some cancers.

Fresh, unprocessed vegetable and fruit juices

Pure unprocessed water

6. Spices and Herbs

Basil	Cinnamon	Chili Pepper
Cloves	Cocoa	Licorice
Mint	Oregano	Parsley
Rosemary	Thyme	Turmeric

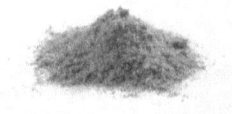

7. Seeds and Nuts

Almonds	Hazelnuts	Linseed
Pecans	Sunflower seeds	Walnuts

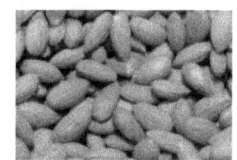

8. Herbs also have anti-inflammatory and anti-oxidant nutrients.

Turmeric: Turmeric extract is effective against all sorts of inflammatory disorders and is the first one chosen among herbs for the treatment of inflammatory medical disorders. For example, those suffering from arthritis or tendonitis have immensely benefited from as little as 200 milligrams of Turmeric three times a day. Turmeric contains helenalin, a powerful anti-inflammatory nutrient.

Ginger: 500mg to 1000 mg of dry and powdered ginger acts as an awesome natural anti-inflammatory medication if administered for a span same as turmeric. No contraindications have been recorded so far, except that too much of it may produce a burning sensation to the tongue or in the stomach for a limited period.

Boswellin contains Boswellin a general anti-inflammatory for common rheumatoid disorders except for those involving the joints. Boswellin is highly effective against achy pain, tenderness and muscle stiffness.

Whenever someone takes all the above 3 herbs in combination, together they provide very strong anti-inflammatory and warming effects. The warming effects are helpful for improving blood circulation. And good circulation is known to help the healing process as the blood carries nutrients.

On the contrary, the poor circulation can make the pain and discomfort get worse...these combined herbs for inflammation have been used to treat inflammation and pain related conditions as bursitis, sport injuries, osteoarthritis with poor blood circulation (spinal wear and tear) and joint inflammation conditions (rheumatoid arthritis).

If inflammation is a good thing, why do we need anti-inflammatory nutrients?

Because out of control inflammation can becomes a chronic disorder and damage healthy areas in the body. Examples include arthritis of the joints and thickening and stiffening of blood vessel walls.

It can affect individual parts of the body (nose, lung, skin, etc.) or affect the body as a whole (diabetes, heart disease, Parkinson's disease and Alzheimer's).

Some people are more at risk of developing diabetes, etc. because it is found frequently in family members and relatives (genetic).

Note- It is often quoted, "we are what we eat", so watch what you eat. There is no better way than to include the anti-inflammatory and anti-oxidant food nutrients in your daily diet to ensure a happy healthy disease free long life.

Denise Marks, M.D.

Foods Containing Anti-Inflammatory and Anti-oxidant Nutrients Are Considered Anti-Aging Foods as well as Natural Medicines!

Foods containing Anti-inflammatory nutrients are the key to living a longer and healthier life. Basically, inflammation is a normal and essential part of our body's defense system. It is a natural way in which our body reacts to an infection, irritation or other injury.

Also, inflammation refers to a set of biological processes involving the natural reaction of our body to harmful stimuli, i.e. injuries, infections, free radicals, toxins, etc.

Inflammation is the body's attempt at healing or repairing the damage caused by the harmful foreign agents. It does this by removing the harmful stimuli, i.e., irritants, pathogens (agents of infection) and even damaged cells.

Exposure to any of the above mentioned stimuli is basically inevitable in our daily lives. However, our body's natural defense can fight those harmful (toxic) agents to some extent on its own. Anti-inflammatory foods help our body prevent and/or fight against most of the metabolic medical diseases.

Signs and symptoms of the damage caused by inflammation are swelling redness increased temperature, pain, tumors and damaged receptors that do not work properly (i.e., insulin resistance is the result of damaged receptors).

If there aren't enough anti-inflammatory food nutrients consumed to correct the damage caused by this most often necessary biological response to foreign substances, then some or all of the symptoms above can increase to the point of causing cancer and death.

Inflammation basically can be acute (short term) or chronic (long term). Acute inflammation is a sign that the body is trying to heal itself and last within a 24 hour period of time.

Chronic inflammation refers to what happens in our body over a longer period of time. Chronic long term damage happens when our body's natural defenses (mainly our immune system, digestive system, cardiovascular system, etc.) are overwhelmed by the continuous exposure to harmful stimuli, which then renders our body and its natural defenses weak and unable to fight, correct or prevent further damage and disease.

Some examples of most of the common chronic metabolic medical disorders caused by inflammation are: Arthritis, Dermatitis, Gastrointestinal disorders, Neurological disorders, Cardiovascular disorders (Hypertension, Hypercholesterolemia, Hypertriglyceridemia, Atherosclerosis, Angina, Heart Attack, Stroke, etc.), Chronic Renal (Kidney) disorders, some Eye diseases, Diabetes, Obesity, Inflammatory Bowel Diseases, some Cancers, Aging Processes, and Auto-Immune diseases (those diseases that result when our body's defense mechanisms start attacking itself).

APPENDIX #4 THE GLYCEMIC INDEX OF FOODS

Extremely High-Glycemic Foods: Corn flakes, potatoes, honey, rice (instant or whole grain), rice cereal, sweet bread - especially French and other sweet rolls, Cookies, Cake (if frosted), Candies.

THE GLYCEMIC STANDARD - IS WHITE BREAD - (made with enriched white flour) - if the label says whole wheat but the first item listed is enriched white flour the wheat germ (the good healthy stuff) has been removed.

High-Glycemic Foods: Bread (rye, or stone ground whole wheat) Cereals (Grape Nuts, Muesli, Shredded Wheat, Cheerios, Raisin Bran and of course all extra sweetened cereals), Corn, Orange juice, Grape juice, Apricots (dried), Banana, Mango, Raisins, Papaya, Crackers, Tortilla, Brown Rice, Candy bars, Cookies, Corn chips, Potato chips, Ice Cream, Fruit pies, Cake.

Moderately High-Glycemic Foods: Buckwheat, Pumpernickel bread, Macaroni, Yams, Green peas, All Bran cereal, Bulgur, Spaghetti, Sweet potatoes, Baked Beans (canned), Fruit cocktail, Pears (canned), Oatmeal cookies, Sponge cake, Kidney beans (canned), Pineapple juice, Apple Juice, Cranberry juice, Grapes, and Grape juice.

Moderately Low -Glycemic Foods: White beans, Green peas (dried), Butter beans, Kidney beans, Black beans, Black-eyed peas, Lima beans, Chickpeas (garbanzo), Tomato soup, Yogurt, Orange, Pears, Apple, Milk, Grapefruit juice (unsweetened), some Nuts.

Low-Glycemic Foods: Barley, Red Lentils, Grapefruit, Peach, Soybeans, Plums, Peanuts, Fructose, Most Nuts. Fructose by-passes the Pancreas and goes straight to the Liver to be made into **ketone bodies** for energy first and if not used for energy will be converted into fats.

NOTE- LOW GLYCEMIC, COMPLEX CARBOHYDRATES ARE ALMOST ALWAYS ASSOCIATED WITH <u>HIGH FIBER CONTENT</u> - WHICH IS A GOOD THING.

The "glycemic index" is a measure of how quickly a given carbohydrate is converted to glucose and/or fructose (i.e., simple sugars) for energy and how much and how quickly they affect insulin levels. <u>Each food (carbohydrate) is assigned a numbered rating</u>. The lower the rating, the slower the digestion and absorption of that carbohydrate will be. Slower digestion and absorption of food nutrients is good. That is because this slow distribution of nutrients will not cause the pancreas to release a surge of insulin. Another way of stating this fact is that low glycemic carbohydrates provide a more gradual, healthier infusion of sugars and therefore lower insulin levels in the bloodstream.

On the other hand, a high rating means that blood-glucose levels are increased quickly, which stimulates the pancreas to secrete a surge of insulin for the purpose of quickly dropping this <u>higher than normal</u> blood-sugar level back to normal. <u>These rapid fluctuations of blood-sugar and insulin levels are not healthy. These rapid fluctuations of blood sugar and insulin levels cause internal damage to cell structures and the cells themselves.</u> The first noticeable damage is to the insulin receptors. Second these rapid fluctuations of blood sugar and insulin levels triggers an imbalance that effects unhealthy changes with other hormones and enzymes (protein) that control many of the necessary metabolic processes in the body. .

An influx of sugar into the bloodstream upsets the body's blood-sugar balance, triggering the release of excessive amounts of insulin. Sugar (glucose) raises the blood insulin level rapidly and higher than any of the low glycemic complex carbohydrates.

Note- Carbohydrates that cause a rapid increase in blood sugar are known as simple carbohydrates or carbohydrates with a high

glycemic index. Carbohydrates are metabolized slowly and yield a gradual rise of blood sugar are known as complex carbohydrates or carbohydrates with a low glycemic index.

High-glycemic Foods. Foods with a high glycemic index (sugar) stimulate the pancreas to secrete a surge of insulin. Believe it or not, this actually causes low blood sugar because the high insulin level causes the blood sugar to drop too quickly. And symptoms including hyper-activity, a decreased attention span and learning difficulties and even syncope spells with seizure like activity - will result. This extremely fast drop in blood sugar is then corrected by the liver where a process called glycogenolysis is triggered to occur in which stored glycogen is converted into glucose to at least temporarily correct the blood glucose level.

Foods with a high glycemic index initially cause the blood sugar to shoot up. But then this rise in blood sugar signals the pancreas that the body has too much sugar. The pancreas then secretes a surge of insulin to bring the blood sugar level back down. This excessive release of insulin actually causes the blood sugar to become too low.

High glycemic foods are any of the following: i.e., processed starches (especially starches that are ground, puffed, flaked, rolled or beat into submission) such as white bread made with enriched white flour, rice cakes and white rice and even potatoes whether -instant, fried, baked or mashed. Eating these foods is basically the same as eating candy as far as your body and brain are concerned.

Remember, low-glycemic foods (complex carbohydrates) do not cause excessive amounts of insulin to flood into your body. Therefore, your blood sugar remains more stable without the highs and lows. You will find it easier to focus and learn when provided with low-glycemic carbohydrates.

It is easy to see that simply avoiding sweets (sugars) in your diet is not enough. Limiting or avoiding all high-glycemic foods is the key to the prevention of these deadly metabolic medical diseases. The more you are able to regulate your blood sugar and insulin, the better you brain will be able to work or learn new tasks. Also, the better your chances are - that you will be able to control your weight and prevent diabetes as well as prevent elevated cholesterol, triglyceride and high blood pressure the lead to or cause heart problems. This is because insulin affects the way your body processes both carbohydrates and fat (triglycerides/cholesterol).

Note- It is often quoted, "we are what we eat", so watch what you eat.

There is no better way than to include the anti-inflammatory and anti-oxidant food nutrients in your daily diet to ensure a happy healthy disease free long life.

Biography - Denise Oldenberg Marks, M.D.

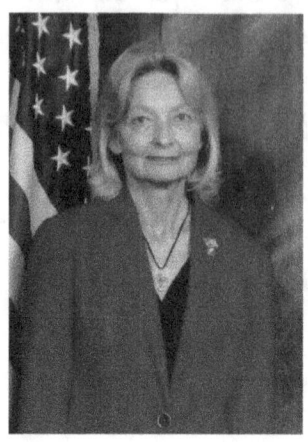

Denise is a retired medical doctor who has renewed her interest in writing. She specializes in subjects related to medicine, nutrition, safe and effective means of weight loss. After more than 20 years as a practicing family physician, she has retired to the Mountain Home area of Arkansas to begin a "physician guided weight loss program" that focuses on good nutrition and healthy life style changes that will be beneficial in not only correcting health problems but will also help individuals achieve their ideal weight and a healthier life style and therefore prevent many of today's age-related metabolic medical diseases.

Born in Billings, Montana, Denise graduated in 1965 from Huntley Project High School in Worden, Montana. She then joined the U.S. Marine Corps and served her country from 1965 – 1968. After finishing her military obligation she used the GI Bill to obtain a college education. She received her BS degree in Health and Physical Education with a minor in Chemistry and Biology and began teaching high school science in 1971. She taught school for 7 years in Louisiana. However, when one of her students was accepted into medical school, she realized she could also become a medical doctor. She enjoyed teaching but wanted to help people, one-on-one, with the knowledge she had gained. As a classroom teacher with class sizes of 24 to 30 students: she felt she was more of a disciplinarian than a teacher.

Denise received her M.D. degree in 1986 from Louisiana State University Medical Center in Shreveport, La. In 1988 she received her Arkansas medical license and then moved to Arkansas where she began her medical practice in rural Arkansas, between Dover and Witt Springs. She also worked as an Emergency Room Physician in various small hospitals throughout northern Arkansas from 1995 to 2003. In 1998 she moved her medical practice to the Salem, Horseshoe Bend and the Cherokee Village area of Arkansas where she not only kept her clinic opened but continued to work in the Salem and Cherokee Village Hospitals as one of their ER physicians. She also delivered babies at the Salem hospital from 1998 until 2002. This was during the (time) when rural hospitals could obtain malpractice insurance for family physicians doing obstetrics as well as a time that family physicians could afford malpractice in obstetrics.

Her mission still remains "to serve others" by teaching or instructing them on how they can become a healthier individual by using natural (food) nutrients. She believes good nutrition and a healthy weight are at the core of achieving this goal for all individuals. By achieving a healthy weight and eating healthy (food) nutrients, (avoiding sugar, nonnutritive artificial sweeteners and hydrogenated oils or trans-fats, i.e., margarine and shortening and processed foods made with these "trans-fats"), she believes individuals can prevent, treat and even cure many of their own health problems. For example, stress management and poor nutritional eating are known to be risk factors that contribute to anxiety, arthritis, diabetes, hypertension, heart disease due to high cholesterol/high triglyceride eye disease, depression, acid reflux (GERD), neurological diseases and chronic pain issues, etc. Knowledge, about good nutrition and safe and effective weight loss as well as how to handle stress, will be the center of focus at each encounter.

Denise is the proud and happy mother of 2 adult children and a grandmother. In fact she wants to dedicate this book to her two sons, Jason and Justin Sharbono, who sacrificed the time she spent away studying to become a medical doctor. Also, Denise is a proud Marine and a member of Twin Lakes Marine and the Marine Corps League. As a veteran of the Vietnam era she continues to help veterans, through diet, counseling and medication, who deal with post traumatic issues and depression, overcome some of the issues that hinder them from achieving a better quality of life.